Retirement Communities

An American Original

Retirement Communities
An American Original

Michael E. Hunt, Allan G. Feldt,
Robert W. Marans, Leon A. Pastalan,
and Kathleen L. Vakalo

The Haworth Press
New York

Retirement Communities: An American Original has also been published as *Journal of Housing for the Elderly*, Volume 1, Numbers 3/4, Winter 1983.

The Haworth Press, Inc., 28 East 22 Street, New York, NY 10010

Library of Congress Cataloging in Publication Data
Main entry under title:

Retirement communities.

    "Also . . . published as Journal of housing for the elderly, volume 1, numbers 3/4, Winter 1983"—
    Bibliography: p.
    1. Retirement communities—United States—Case studies. 2. Life care communities—United States—Case studies. I. Hunt, Michael E.
HQ1063.R47 1984   307.7   83-26506
ISBN 0-86656-267-2

Retirement Communities: An American Original

Journal of Housing for the Elderly
Volume 1, Numbers 3/4

CONTENTS

Contributors

Allan G. Feldt received his Ph.D. in Sociology from The University of Michigan, and taught Urban Sociology and City Planning at Cornell University for nine years. Returning to Michigan in 1971, he has been engaged in research and teaching primarily in Urban and Regional Planning. His current research interests include decentralism, energy planning, and simulation/gaming. Recent publications include chapters in *Housing for a Maturing Population*, edited by Eric Smart; *The Planner's Use of Information*, edited by Hemalata Dandekar; and *Energy Management in Local and State Parks*, with Mitchell Rycus et al.

Michael E. Hunt is an assistant professor in the Environment, Textiles and Design Program at the University of Wisconsin-Madison. He teaches courses concerning the relationship of the designed environment and human behavior and is conducting environmental learning research. He received a Doctor of Architecture Degree as well as a Specialist in Aging Certificate from The University of Michigan. He holds a Master of Regional and Community Planning from Kansas State University and a Bachelor of Arts in Architecture from the University of Arkansas.

Robert W. Marans is a professor in the College of Architecture and Urban Planning at The University of Michigan and a research scientist at the University's Institute for Social Research. He also serves on the Executive Committee of the Ph.D. program in Urban, Environmental, and Technological Planning and is a senior research fellow at the Brookdale Institute of Gerontology and Adult Human Development in Jerusalem. Dr. Marans' research interests focus on the concept and measurement of neighborhood quality, high-rise living for the elderly, and environmental evaluation. He is the recipient of a 1982 Applied Research Award for *Progressive Architecture* and a 1983 award for design research excellence from the National Endowment for the Arts.

Leon A. Pastalan, Ph.D., received his Ph.D. from Syracuse University and is currently Chairman of the Doctoral Program in Architecture, The University of Michigan. He is also Director of the National Policy Center on Housing. Professor Pastalan is a researcher of long standing in the field of environments for the elderly, with an emphasis in several areas, including sensory deficits, spatial behavior, and housing relocation. He is the author/editor of many books and national publications resulting from his work, including most recently, *Environmental Context of Aging: Life-Styles, Environment Quality and Living Arrangements* (1979) with Byerts and Howell and *Man Environment Reference 2* (MER 2), 1983.

Kathleen L. Vakalo was born in Wausatosa, Wisconsin. She received her undergraduate degree in Philosophy and her master's in Educational Psychology from The University of Michigan, Ann Arbor. Her research work has been in developmental psychology and gerontology. She is currently working in development at The University of Michigan.

Foreword

Housing is intimately related to every nuance of community life. Because it is the major source of revenue for local governments, housing is also the major reason for expenditures by them. It is the pivot on which turn the location and character of community facilities and services, all of them expensive to install, expensive to maintain, and expensive to change. When the character of the supply and demand for housing forces shifts in land use, the community must adjust this complex of services and facilities to different levels of use. Such a shift is occurring presently in many areas across this country through the emergence of the retirement community, a new life-style generated by the special housing and other environmental needs of an ever-increasing aging population.

Retirement communities have been brought to fruition by a variety of sponsors including fraternal lodges, labor unions, religious groups, voluntary associations, and real estate developers. Many of these settlements have developed, practically speaking, an autonomous community life while others depend in part or in whole on the services of the outside community. Each type of community involves certain gains and losses to the individual with respect to security, responsibility, freedom, and privacy.

Whatever one may make of the retirement community movement there is an increasing proportion of Americans who are confronted by the empty-nest and compulsory retirement. Increasingly they are able, financially and otherwise, to enter the housing market for specialized housing commensurate with their needs, a trend which will insure investment in retirement housing. To be sure, many and perhaps most people in this category will find housing other than in retirement communities. Nevertheless, there will be in the future as there are now, many elderly households demanding to have their very particular housing preferences satisfied by highly specialized packages of housing and services. These specialized packages will be directed toward meeting the elderly's preferences for independence, self-determination, privacy, health maintenance, companionship of peers, security, and meaningful work-substitutes which have not been available to date in the typical community.

There are currently well over a million older adults living in some type of planned residential setting. This book focuses on the wide variety of retirement communities in the United States. Representative case histories of these communities are examined in terms of how change over time has affected their function and character and what the future may hold for them and for us.

Leon A. Pastalan
Editor

Introduction

It seems indisputable that retirement communities have established themselves in the United States as a viable housing option for older people. What is disputable, however, is a clear understanding of what is meant by the term "retirement community." This lack of a consensus definition has resulted in a rather fragmented body of knowledge about retirement communities. It has thus been difficult to develop a general understanding of how retirement communities are planned and developed, how they evolve, and how they meet the needs and capabilities of older people of various ages and circumstances.

In a national study on which this book is based,* we have defined retirement communities quite broadly so as not to exclude potentially significant retirement housing options open to older people. To make our broad perspective of retirement communities meaningful, it must be possible to classify the communities in a manner which reflects their similarities and differences. It is this logic which fostered the development of our typology. A typology makes it possible to compare the development and experiences of a wide range of retirement communities on a comparative basis. Such analyses should shed insight into the relative strengths and weaknesses of various types of retirement communities with respect to the varying needs, capabilities, and desires of older people.

To develop and illustrate our typology, we have organized this book as a series of ten case studies which examine a wide range of retirement communities in depth. While we analyzed eighteen communities, it was felt that the selection of two representative cases for each community type would be sufficient to provide the necessary in-depth profile without exhausting the reader and at the same time avoiding unnecessary redundancy. These case studies are preceded by a review of the retirement community literature and a discussion of how we have defined and classified retirement communities into a multi-dimensional typology. The case studies are followed by a

*Administration on Aging, U.S. Department of Health and Human Services, Grant Number 90AR-0011/02.

summary chapter which synthesizes the experiences and characteristics of all eighteen communities we investigated. Thus, we feel this
book represents a resource which can be used to study individual
retirement communities in depth, and/or to study the similarities and
differences among retirement communities with respect to the typology we have developed.

Michael E. Hunt
Allan G. Feldt
Robert W. Marans
Leon A. Pastalan
Kathleen L. Vakalo

Retirement Communities

An American Original

Chapter 1

The Retirement
Community Phenomenon

Retirement Community Research: A Review

Retirement communities are not a recent phenomena in the United States. Some date back to the 1920s, when various labor, fraternal, and religious organizations acquired relatively inexpensive property in Florida with the intent of creating a supportive living environment for their retiring members. Moosehaven, for example, was established in 1922 by the Loyal (fraternal) Order of Moose as a means of caring for its retired members while at the same time demonstrating the fraternal claims of the Order (Gottschalk, 1975). Other sponsored communities in Florida were created for benevolent purposes until a series of catastrophes, culminating with the stock market crash of 1929, brought their development to a standstill (Duncan et al., 1978).

The post-World War II period represented a new era of retirement community development, as private builders in Florida and in other parts of the U.S. recognized the potential for marketing homes to a growing population of older Americans. Despite their success in attracting home buyers, planned residential developments catering to relatively homogeneous age groups have been viewed with skepticism by a number of social critics. Margaret Mead characterized such developments as "golden ghettos," while Lewis Mumford argued that such large-scale organized living quarters for older persons were socially unnatural and should be avoided at all costs (Mumford, 1956).

The proliferation of retirement communities during the 1950s was accompanied by a number of studies designed to enhance an understanding of these communities and their residents. While these studies, for the most part, were descriptive in nature and characterized communities according to their population makeup and the

1

types of housing and services they offered, several focused on the activities and sentiments of retirement community residents. In part, efforts were being made to determine if the "health" of retirement communities was as bad as claimed by the social critics. In one early study of life in a retirement community, Hoyt found that most residents (88 percent) preferred to live "in a community such as this, where everyone is retired, rather than one in which people were working" (1954). Reasons given for preferring the age-segregated environment dealt with the possibilities for association with others, mutual assistance in time of illness, and the desirability of being in a quiet, child-free setting. Similar findings were reported by Hamovitch and Larson (1966) in a study of residents of Leisure World, California. The researchers found that three-quarters of the residents had been pleased with their move to the retirement community, and most (87 percent) said they had never considered moving out. In still another retirement community study in central Florida (Aldridge, 1959), a highly supportive environment was preferred by residents who saw this as important to their well-being. Similarly, aged migrants to age-segregated retirement communities in Arizona were found to have higher morale than aged migrants living in nearby age-integrated communities (Bultena & Wood, 1969). More recently, researchers at the University of North Carolina examined residents' attitudes in two retirement communities and compared them with attitudes of older residents in planned new towns. It was concluded that age-segregated communities provide more opportunity for social contact and the avoidance of social isolation than age-integrated new communities or conventional communities occupied by older people (Burby & Weiss, 1976).

The empirical research covering older persons living in "retirement communities" has been conducted in settings ranging from trailer parks and hotels to enclaves containing various housing arrangements and resident support services. Clearly, the term retirement community has taken on different meanings to different scholars. Some consider them to be relatively self-contained small communities, spatially separated from large population centers. Others have used the concept to refer to any communal living arrangement composed entirely or primarily of retired people. Whether or not located in an isolated situation, the distinguishing feature of the place or places under study has been the residents who, for the most part, were not employed or actively engaged in their regular occupation.

One of the first attempts to systematically define retirement communities was made by Webber and Osterbind (1961), who classified retirement housing on the basis of the degree to which it involved congregate, segregate, and/or institutional living. One class of housing was the retirement village, which they described as "a small community relatively independent, segregated, and non-institutional, whose population was mostly older people, separated more or less completely from their regular or career occupations in gainful or non-paid employment." The retirement village is viewed as non-institutional, in the sense that the population is largely free of the regimen imposed by common food, common rules, common quarters, and common authority (1961).

More recent definitions also discuss the concept of independence and a relatively active older population living in a segregated setting. In a study of retirement communities in California, for example, retirement communities were defined as planned, low-density developments of permanent buildings designed to house active adults over the age of 50 and equipped to provide a wide range of services and leisure activities (Barker, 1966). Similarly, a study of retirement communities in New Jersey described them as planned, low-density, age-restricted developments, constructed by private capital, and offering extensive recreational services and relatively low-cost housing for purchase (Heintz, 1976). Lawton (1980) classifies retirement communities as one form of planned housing for the elderly and characterizes them as privately developed, self-contained places which impose an age limitation on its residents and which contain purchased homes and shopping, medical, and active leisure services. The Lawton and other definitions share several features. The practice of age segregation is noted in all, but the degree to which a community is segregated by age may vary. Some definitions imply absolute segregation, while others state that residents are *mainly* older people. All definitions suggest that retirement community residents are physically well and active and some may even be engaged in part-time or full-time employment. Finally, the concept of a planned or intentional community for older people is imbedded in each definition.

Despite commonalities, retirement communities as discussed in the literature vary with respect to inclusiveness. Some consider community attributes such as size, intensity of development, sponsorship, levels of service, tenure arrangements for residents, and location, while others ignore these attributes as part of their description.

With such diversity, it has been suggested that rather than relying on a single definition of retirement communities, a classification system or typology is needed in order to better describe this particular living arrangement for the elderly.

More than 20 years ago, Burgess (1961) classified retirement communities according to their sponsorship, location, the type of services they offered, and their housing design. Others have described retirement communities according to their size, financial arrangements, type of architecture, and provision for leisure activities. Heintz (1976), for example, states that housing for older people can be differentiated according to the degree to which it promotes autonomy for the residents and opportunities for social interaction through work and leisure activities. Webber and Osterbind (1961) classify retirement villages according to three groupings: real estate developments; supervised planned communities; and full-care homes and communities. Supervised and planned communities are further classified as trailer parks, dispersed dwelling communities, and retirement hotels.

There appears to be as much variation in the classification of retirement communities as there is in attempts to define them. Some classifications are more exclusive than others, and rarely has a type of community within any classification system been clearly specified as to the boundaries or limits of what living arrangement would be considered within it. Furthermore, retirement communities have been treated as static environments, with no provision made for considering their dynamic nature. As with all residential developments, retirement communities and the populations within them change over time; communities grow in size; their physical structures and populations age; and new services to support the aging populations are introduced while others are curtailed or eliminated. It seems appropriate then to consider new ways of defining and classifying retirement communities which are more precise than definitions, and which take into account changes in population, size, and the nature of development.

A Broader Perspective

As stated earlier, we have defined retirement communities quite broadly. We view retirement communities as being aggregations of housing units and at least a minimal level of services planned for older people who are predominantly healthy and retired. In essence, three criteria are considered in our broad definition: housing, services, and residents.

It should be noted that our definition places no stipulations on housing design or tenure arrangements. Thus, both a single high-rise building with rental apartments and a complete new town offering home ownership qualify in the housing component of our definition.

The service component of the definition is not as clear-cut. We feel that for a development to be a community, there must be at least some common service provided for the residents. Otherwise, the development is merely a collection of independent living units.

The residents form the final component of the definition. Our definition stipulates that at least half of the residents must be over 50 years of age and that no more than half of the residents can be in need of nursing care. Thus, age-integrated communities are included in our definition and communities which house residents of whom most need nursing care are excluded. The health restriction is intended to exclude nursing homes or similar facilities from our definition.

Two other criteria often mentioned in definitions of retirement communities are not included in ours: sponsorship and work status of residents. According to our definition, retirement communities can be built under various forms of sponsorship and may house older people still engaged in labor market activity.

As part of our study of retirement communities, we also compiled a comprehensive listing of retirement communities (Feldt et al., 1981). The listing reflects our definition plus two further restrictions. First, only communities with a population of at least 100 residents were included. This restriction was imposed to help manage such an undertaking. Secondly, communities which are actually managed or governed by governmental agencies were excluded. This was done in accordance with the wishes of our funding agency.[1] Utilizing our broad definition and the two additional restrictions, nearly 2,400 retirement communities were identified with a total population of nearly one million people in the late 1970s. This means that the total population of retirement communities, as we have broadly defined them, represents less than 5 percent of older people in the U.S. Nevertheless, the fact that nearly one mil-

---

[1]The research on which this book is based was funded by the Administration on Aging, U.S. Department of Health and Human Services.

lion older people have made the decision to live in this highly specialized form of housing development emphasizes the need to better understand their characteristics and experiences.

Selection of Retirement Communities to Study

The selection of retirement communities to study in detail followed the principle of maximizing differences among communities while minimizing travel. The first step of this procedure was to identify regions of the country containing high concentrations of retirement communities (target regions). This accomplished two things: first, it reduced the number of retirement communities from which to choose; and second, it identified concentrations of communities which would enable us to make regional comparisons.

Four target regions were identified. One consisted of southern California (Los Angeles area) and Arizona (Phoenix area). A second target region was central Florida, including the Tampa Bay area and Orlando. The northeast United States including New York, New Jersey, and Maryland was selected as another region. The fourth target region was identified in the midwest states of Illinois, Michigan, and Ohio.

The next step of the selection process involved classifying the retirement communities in the target regions with respect to six attributes: building type, population, recreation facilities, health care facilities, sponsorship/developer type, and opening date. In addition to these characteristics, priority was also given to those retirement communities for which written material, including quantitive data, were available.

Building types were divided into three groups: 1) cluster housing which includes large multi-dwelling unit buildings, 2) detached housing which includes single-family homes and two, three, or four plexes, and 3) mobile homes.

The population of retirement communities was also categorized into three groups: large communities housing over 5,000 residents; medium-sized communities with 1,000 to 5,000 residents; and small communities with fewer than 1,000 residents.

Recreation facilities were categorized as either extensive or limited. Given the incomplete sources describing retirement communities available to us at that time, no attempt was made to further classify recreation facilities as being either active or passive, and indoor or outdoor. Recreation facilities were considered extensive if the original source mentioned a swimming pool, golf course(s), or tennis courts. The lack of these facilities constituted limited recreation facilities.

It was not possible to describe the medical or health care facilities beyond stating whether or not they were noted in the description of the community in published sources. Thus, the categories for health care facilities were merely "yes" and "no."

Sponsorship of retirement communities was investigated at two levels. First, we categorized sponsors/developers as being profit or non-profit. In addition, we sought to compare and contrast the development strategies and philosophies of various major for-profit developers. To do so, we compared the retirement communities of different developers in the same region, and those developed by the same developer in different regions. This strategy allowed us to ascertain both developer and regional differences in retirement communities. Three major developers were considered in this manner: Leisure Technology Corporation, Rossmoor Corporation, and Del E. Webb Development Company.

The age of retirement communities was also considered in our selection process. We attempted to select communities which had existed for relatively long and for short periods of time. In this way, we could compare communities which had evolved over time to those which were relatively young and in the early stages of a similar evolutionary process.

After classifying the various characteristics of retirement communities in the target regions, a list of typical communities from each region was developed. This list was used to select a sample of communities that was generally representative of each target region in the country. In addition, our sample was weighted to roughly represent the regional distribution of retirement communities, i.e., more in the California/Arizona and Florida regions than the Midwest and Northeast regions.

A list of the retirement communities selected and visited, together with their key attributes is presented in Table 1.1.

A Typology of Retirement Communities

As a result of our detailed study of all 18 retirement communities, we have devised a typology of retirement communities. This task was complicated by the fact that retirement communities do not separate neatly into mutually exclusive groups when considering their

TABLE 1.1

CHARACTERISTICS OF RETIREMENT COMMUNITIES VISITED

RETIREMENT COMMUNITY	REGION	BUILDING TYPE	SIZE	RECREATION FACILITIES AVAILABLE?	MEDICAL FACILITIES AVAILABLE?	SPONSOR TYPE	OPENING DATE
1) Baptist Gardens Long Beach, Cal.	Cal./Ariz.	Cluster	Small	Limited	No	Non-Profit	1975
2) Country Village Apartments Mira Loma, Cal.	Cal./Ariz.	Cluster	Medium	Extensive	No	Profit	1966
3) Leisure Village Camarillo, Cal.	Cal./Ariz.	Detached	Medium	Extensive	No	Profit (Leisure Technology Corporation)	1973
4) Leisure World Laguna Hills, Cal.	Cal./Ariz.	Detached	Large	Extensive	Yes	Profit	1964
5) Riviera Mobile Home Park Scottsdale, Ariz.	Cal./Ariz.	Mobile Home	Small	Limited	No	Profit (Rosamoor Corp.)	1964
6) Sun City Arizona	Cal./Ariz.	Detached	Large	Extensive	Yes	Profit (Del E. Webb Development Co.)	1960
7) Friendship Village Schaumburg, Ill.	Midwest	Cluster	Small	Limited	Yes	Non-Profit	1977
8) Otterbein Home Near Lebanon, Ohio	Midwest	Cluster	Small	Limited	Yes	Non-Profit	1913
9) Presbyterian Home Evansville, Ill.	Midwest	Detached and Cluster	Small	Limited	Yes	Non-Profit	1914

TABLE 1.1 (continued)

	Region	Housing Type	Size	Services		Status	Year
10) Leisure Village West, Ocean County, N.J.	Northeast	Detached	Medium	Extensive	No	Profit (Leisure Technology Corporation)	1972
11) Leisure World, Montgomery County, Md.	Northeast	Detached and Cluster	Medium	Extensive	Yes	Profit (Rossmoor Corp.)	1966
12) Williams Memorial Residence, New York, N.Y.	Northeast	Cluster	Small	Limited	No	Non-Profit	1969
13) Bradenton Trailer Park, Bradenton	Florida	Mobile Home	Medium	Limited	No	Non-Profit	1936
14) Hawthorne, Leesburg	Florida	Mobile Home	Medium	Extensive	No	Profit	1973
15) Orange Gardens, Kissimmee	Florida	Detached	Medium	Limited	No	Profit	1954
16) Sun City Center, Near Tampa	Florida	Detached	Large	Extensive	Yes	Profit (originally Del E. Webb Development Company)	1960
17) Sunny Shores Villas, St. Petersburg	Florida	Cluster	Small	Limited	Yes	Non-Profit	1954
18) Trailer Estates, Bradenton	Florida	Mobile Home	Medium	Limited	No	Profit	1955

many characteristics. Furthermore, any or all of the characteristics can change over time. Consequently, we have devised a multi-dimensional typology which permits the different genre of retirement communities to be compared and contrasted along four major attributes, each of which may be dimensioned. The four attributes are as follows: 1) the scale of the community; 2) the characteristics of the population; 3) the kinds and amounts of services offered; and 4) the sponsorship or auspices under which the community was built.

This typology makes it possible to conceptually view retirement communities as dynamic entities having specific features, any of which can be altered by planned change or the passage of time. For example, one retirement community may grow in size, and, with an increase in population, expand the number and types of recreational and social services. In another retirement community planned for a relatively young and active population, more supportive health care may be required as the residents age chronologically. Having a multi-dimensional typology makes it possible to identify and trace the patterns of change in retirement communities along dimensions of each major attribute.

The first attribute of scale refers to the size of the retirement community population. The same size categories are used as in the retirement community selection process described earlier: large retirement communities contain populations of more than 5,000 residents; medium-sized retirement communities house 1,000 to 5,000 residents; small retirement communities contain less than 1,000 residents. As we noted earlier, we have identified nearly 2,400 retirement communities, housing nearly one million residents. Most (96 percent) communities are small, containing less than 1,000 people; only about one retirement community in a hundred has a population of 5,000 or more residents.

The second attribute, characteristics of the retirement community population, is defined by the health and age of residents and consists of three dimensions (see Figure 1.1). One dimension is made up of retirees who, for the most part, are healthy and no older than 75. A second dimension consists of retirees who tend to be older than 75 years of age and generally in good health. The third dimension includes a mix of predominantly older retirees (75 years or older) who are both healthy and frail. Elderly residents who live together and are predominantly frail are likely to be found in nursing homes, a living arrangement excluded from our definition of retirement com-

Figure 1.1
Population Attribute

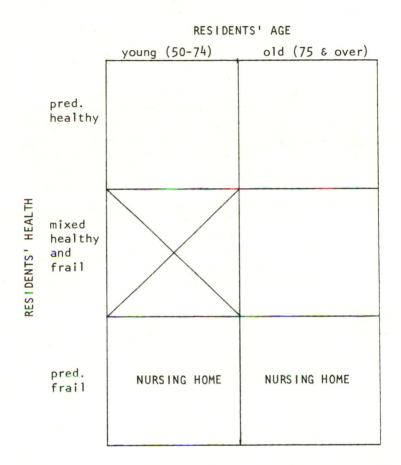

munities. Similarly, we believe that places housing a mix of both healthy and frail retirees who are predominantly young (50-74) are rare and were thus excluded as a dimension.

The service attribute of retirement communities considers the type and quantity of health, recreational/leisure, and commercial services and facilities available to residents. Facilities and services related to health care can include hospitals, nursing homes, clinics, doctors' offices, or special home care programs. Outdoor recreation facilities include golf courses, tennis courts, marinas, and swimming pools, whereas indoor facilities range from meeting rooms to club houses and libraries. Programs such as arts and crafts, classes, and outings to local area attractions are also considered. Commercial services vary from shopping centers with an array of stores to a gift shop, or a privately operated snack bar in a single building housing elderly retirees. We consider health care and outdoor recreation to be the most important aspects of the service attribute. For purposes of building our typology, other services (social programs and facilities, commercial, housekeeping, maintenance) are combined. Dimensioning of the service attribute is shown in Figure 1.2.

Finally, two types of sponsors or developers of retirement communities are considered in the typology: one is the building or development company that plans and builds a retirement community as a profit-making venture; the other is the non-profit sponsor such as a church group, fraternal order, or union.

When dimensions of the four attributes are considered simultaneously, it becomes clear that any combination of them can be used to classify a retirement community (see Figure 1.3). Moreover, the attributes of one or more dimensions in any community can change over time, e.g., the residents may become increasingly frail, the population may grow in size, community sponsorship may change, and so forth. Hence, a multi-dimensional typology which takes into account the changing nature of retirement communities was viewed as essential to understanding them.

In considering the dimensions of the four attributes in relationship to our broad definition of retirement communities, five types or classes are proposed: retirement new towns, retirement villages, retirement subdivisions, retirement residences, and continuing care retirement centers. A brief characterization of each follows.

Retirement New Town

A new town is a large retirement community having various health care services and an extensive network of outdoor recreational facilities and leisure programs designed primarily for retirees. It also contains at least a moderate amount of commercial and business uses. For the most part, new towns are the creation of private developers and are marketed for young, active retirees. Although only one percent of the retirement communities in the United States

Figure 1.2
Service Attribute

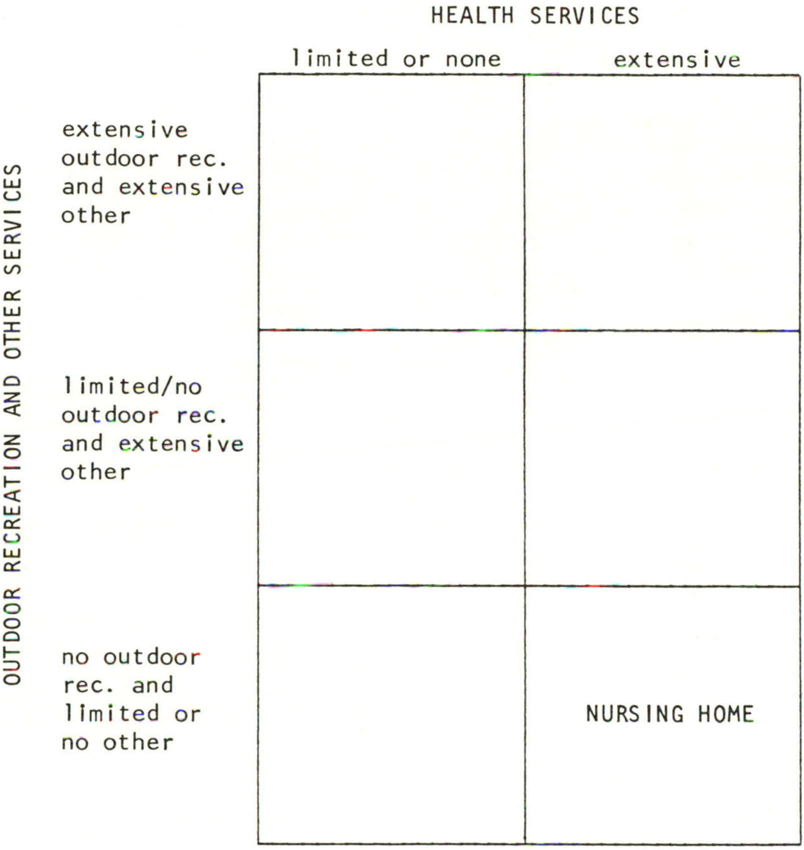

HEALTH SERVICES

limited or none   extensive

OUTDOOR RECREATION AND OTHER SERVICES

extensive outdoor rec. and extensive other

limited/no outdoor rec. and extensive other

no outdoor rec. and limited or no other

NURSING HOME

are new towns, they house about 30 percent of the entire retirement community population.[2]

[2]It should be noted that these estimates and those which follow are based on data from only two-thirds (64 percent) of the 2,363 retirement communities listed in our directory. In one-third of the communities, information covering the availability of medical facilities, sponsorship, or size was not available and, therefore, a community classification could not be assigned.

Figure 1.3

ATTRIBUTES	DIMENSIONS		
	large	medium	small
SCALE			
RESIDENT CHARACTERISTICS	young, predominantly healthy	old, predominantly healthy	old, mixed healthy and frail
LEVEL OF SERVICES	extensive health, outdoor rec., & other / limited/no health; extensive outdoor rec., & other	limited/no health, outdoor rec., & other / limited/no health, outdoor rec.; extensive other	extensive health; limited outdoor rec.; extensive other
SPONSORSHIP	profit		non-profit

Retirement Village

A retirement village is characterized as a medium-sized community and, as in the case of the new town, features a variety of outdoor recreational facilities and leisure programs. It contains limited commercial facilities, and, if health care is available, it is sparse and unobtrusive. Most retirement villages are privately developed, although historically, a number have been built under union or church sponsorship. As in the case of the new town, they are likely to be targeted for the relatively young, healthy retiree. According to current estimates, villages represent 11 percent of all retirement communities in the U.S. and house approximately 61,000 people.

Retirement Subdivision

Subdivisions vary in scale and generally have limited outdoor recreational facilities and support services for their residents. In most instances, health care and commercial facilities are non-existent. Development is usually under private sponsorship and residents tend to be young retirees in good health. Despite their being characterized as retirement communities which house a predominantly over-50 population, subdivisions are often age-integrated. Data indicate that retirement subdivisions comprise about 10 percent of the retirement communities and house an estimated 87,000 people.

Retirement Residence

A retirement residence is a small retirement community having facilities and programs enabling residents to engage in an array of sedentary individual and group activities. Few, if any opportunities exist for active outdoor recreational pursuits within the community; health care services and commercial uses are either limited or non-existent. Retirement residences are likely to be developed by non-profit sponsors such as church groups, fraternal orders, or service organizations. In many cases, federal assistance programs are used in the development process so as to enable the residences to accommodate low to moderate income retirees. For the most part, occupants are older retirees with few serious health problems. Residences represented nearly half (47 percent) of all retirement communities in existence in 1977 and contained an estimated population of 174,000 people.

Continuing Care Retirement Center

Continuing care centers are small in size and are characterized by comprehensive health care offered as an integral part of the community. Residents attracted to these communities tend to be old and less physically active. A significant number are considered to be frail. While few if any outdoor recreational opportunities are available, continuing care centers offer numerous programs and facilities for more passive forms of leisure. Development is usually achieved under a non-profit sponsor. About one-third of our retirement community listing is classified as continuing care. These communities contain an estimated population of 124,000 retirees.

These five types are summarized in Figure 1.4 which illustrates the predominant set of characteristics of each type of community. The reader is reminded that irregularities in these patterns are known to exist. For example, we are aware of retirement villages and subdivisions that were built under non-profit sponsorship. Similarly, there are some retirement residences and continuing care retirement centers containing more than 1,000 residents. Nevertheless, most communities in our listing can be categorized according to one of these five types.

It should be re-emphasized that this typology allows for a retirement community to evolve from one classification to another. In this regard, we consider the attributes of scale and services to be critical. For instance, a retirement village may grow in size (to over 5,000 population) and add medical services, thereby changing its status to that of a retirement new town. Or a retirement residence may add a nursing wing in order to service its increasingly aging and frail residents. In doing so, it becomes a continuing care center. By comparison, the sponsor and building-type attributes are not critical in that they do not determine a retirement community's classification; they merely further describe the community.

The case studies that follow are arranged alphabetically within the groupings of our typology. All case studies follow the format shown in the abbreviated outline (see Figure 1.5) and contain detailed information on each retirement community visited. Figure 1.6 illustrates the location of the 18 retirement communities along with their typological designation. For a synthesis of the experiences and characteristics of all 18 retirement communities, readers are referred to the final chapter of this book.

Figure 1.4

RETIREMENT NEW TOWN

Scale	large		medium		small	
Resident Characteristics	young, predominantly healthy		old, predominantly healthy		old, mixed healthy and frail	
Level of Services	extensive health, outdoor rec., & other	limited/no health; extensive outdoor rec. & other	limited/no health, outdoor rec., & other	limited/no health, outdoor rec.; extensive other	extensive health; limited outdoor rec.; extensive other	
Sponsorship	profit			non-profit		

RETIREMENT VILLAGE

Scale	large		medium		small	
Resident Characteristics	young, predominantly healthy		old, predominantly healthy		old, mixed healthy and frail	
Level of Services	extensive health, outdoor rec., & other	limited/no health; extensive outdoor rec. & other	limited/no health, outdoor rec., & other	limited/no health, outdoor rec.; extensive other	extensive health; limited outdoor rec.; extensive other	
Sponsorship	profit			non-profit		

RETIREMENT SUBDIVISION

Scale	large		medium		small	
Resident Characteristics	young, predominantly healthy		old, predominantly healthy		old, mixed healthy and frail	
Level of Services	extensive health, outdoor rec., & other	limited/no health; extensive outdoor rec. & other	limited/no health, outdoor rec., & other	limited/no health, outdoor rec.; extensive other	extensive health; limited outdoor rec.; extensive other	
Sponsorship	profit			non-profit		

RETIREMENT RESIDENCE

Scale	large		medium		small	
Resident Characteristics	young, predominantly healthy		old, predominantly healthy		old, mixed healthy and frail	
Level of Services	extensive health, outdoor rec., & other	limited/no health; extensive outdoor rec. & other	limited/no health, outdoor rec., & other	limited/no health, outdoor rec.; extensive other	extensive health; limited outdoor rec.; extensive other	
Sponsorship	profit			non-profit		

CONTINUING CARE RETIREMENT CENTER

Scale	large		medium		small	
Resident Characteristics	young, predominantly healthy		old, predominantly healthy		old, mixed healthy and frail	
Level of Services	extensive health, outdoor rec., & other	limited/no health; extensive outdoor rec. & other	limited/no health, outdoor rec., & other	limited/no health, outdoor rec.; extensive other	extensive health; limited outdoor rec.; extensive other	
Sponsorship	profit			non-profit		

Figure 1.5

RETIREMENT COMMUNITY (RC)
CASE STUDY OUTLINE (Abbreviated)

I. GENERAL DESCRIPTION

Type of RC, size, sponsorship, location, history

II. PHILOSOPHY/PURPOSE OF RC

III. RESIDENT CHARACTERISTICS

Number; socioeconomic profile (age, employment status, etc.);
length of residence; place of origin; moving out and moving
in; level of involvement of residents inside and outside the RC

IV. HOUSING CHARACTERISTICS

Size and type of dwellings; occupancy status (owns, rents,
monthly fees, life care membership, etc.); costs to
residents; waiting lists?
Plans for the future

V. FACILITIES, SERVICES AND PROGRAMS

Availability inside RC; outside RC; costs to residents; demand
for services and programs; outsiders' use of RC facilities

VI. MEDICAL CARE

Availability inside RC; outside RC; costs of using medical
care facilities to residents; demand for services

VII. OWNERSHIP/MANAGEMENT/GOVERNANCE

Who owns, operates RC?; degree of resident involvement;
relationships with local units of government

VIII. FINANCING

Costs to developer (initial and operations costs); costs to
residents; taxes; sources of revenue for developer (user fees,
memberships, etc.)

IX. MARKETING/PLANS FOR THE FUTURE

Advertising; future growth; master planning?
Prospective impacts (problems) of change

X. IMPACTS OF PAST CHANGE IN RC

Effects of change on RC residents
Effects of change on surrounding area
Effects of change in surrounding area on:
physical structure of RC
residents of RC
management/ownership of RC
services provided by RC

Figure 1.6

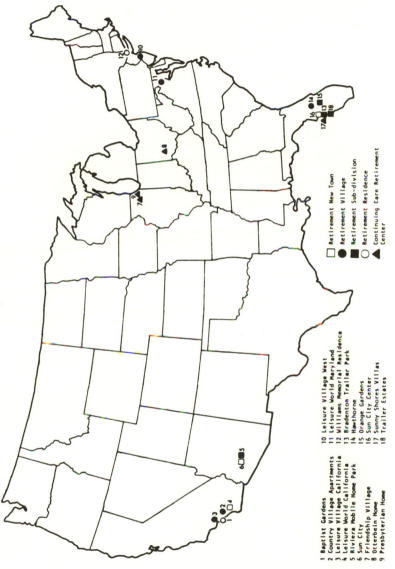

Retirement New Town
Retirement Village
Retirement Sub-division
Retirement Residence
Continuing Care Retirement
Center

1 Baptist Gardens
2 Country Village Apartments
3 Leisure Village California
4 Leisure World California
5 Riviera Mobile Home Park
6 Sun City
7 Friendship Village
8 Otterbein Home
9 Presbyterian Home
10 Leisure Village West
11 Leisure World Maryland
12 Williams Memorial Residence
13 Bradenton Trailer Park
14 Hawthorne
15 Orange Gardens
16 Sun City Center
17 Sunny Shores Villas
18 Trailer Estates

Chapter 2

Retirement New Towns

ROSSMOOR LEISURE WORLD, LAGUNA HILLS, CALIFORNIA

General Description

Rossmoor Leisure World in Laguna Hills (RLWLH) is a "retirement new town" designed for active adults 52 years old or older. It is composed of cooperatives and condominium housing, clustered around open spaces or opening onto courtyards. There are single-family detached, one-, two-, and three-story two to eight plexes, and apartments. It also includes the Towers, a high-rise retirement residence with congregate services. RLWLH offers extensive recreational, medical, security, transportation, and maintenance services. The community opened in 1964 and was developed by the Rossmoor Corporation, an experienced development corporation and the originator of the Leisure World concept.

A site plan of RLWLH is illustrated in Figure 2.1.

Location. Rossmoor Leisure World is located in Laguna Hills, in the Saddleback Valley of Orange County, California. It is halfway between Los Angeles and San Diego, about ten miles southeast of Santa Ana and six miles east of Laguna Beach and the Pacific Coast. Orange County has excellent beaches and harbors, world-renowned recreational facilities such as Disneyland, Knott's Berry Farm, Lion Country Safari, and innumerable parks. The year-round climate is mild. Temperatures range from the mid-40s to the low-80s and average rainfall is 15 inches a year.

Development in north and south Orange County has occurred quite differently. North Orange is older and has followed more traditional patterns of planning, with small residential developments and commercial strip development. There is a balance between housing, commercial, and industrial development as well as a range

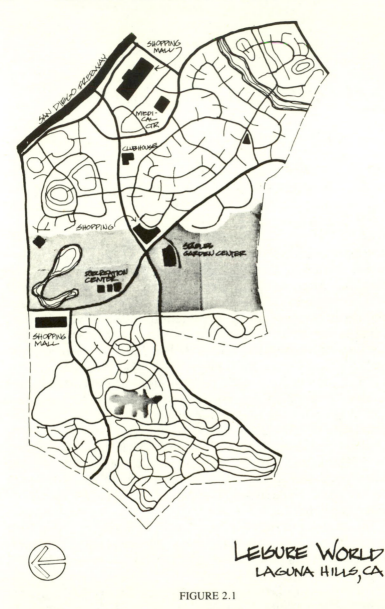

LEISURE WORLD
LAGUNA HILLS, CA

FIGURE 2.1

of housing prices. The north suffers from problems such as traffic congestion, noise pollution, overcrowding, and physical decay.

Development began much later in south Orange, but it was inevitable because of the increasing land costs in Los Angeles County to the north and the pressure of problems in north Orange. Typical development in south Orange has been large parcels of land, phased over time and marketed as communities. RLWLH helped to mold this type of planned community development. The County had never been confronted with a development plan the size or scope of the Rossmoor proposal. The plan included housing, recreation facilities, medical facilities, and complete commercial development and other services normally provided by cities. To accommodate this plan, County officials created a planned community zone. According to one of them, this changed the County's entire approach to planning. The planned community zone allows the developer control of the entire community; it permits cluster housing on smaller lots which creates larger, common areas of green space and it permits multiple land use. However, it also requires prior County approval of both the Master Plan and each detailed section plan.

Subsequent development in south Orange has been in accordance with planned community zoning. According to an assistant director of the Orange County Environmental Management Agency,[1] planned communities have a number of advantages. They have proved viable because of the attention each developer pays both to marketing research and the financial monitoring of the project. This type of planning also reduces the likelihood of the occurrence of the kinds of problems plaguing the north. It has also created a new structure of governance within the County through the homeowners associations which interact with both local and county governments.

Development in south Orange has not been balanced, however. The emphasis has been on housing and commercial development with little attention, until recently, to industry. Housing costs are high and the inexpensive housing needed for employees in industry is not available. These are the problems south Orange must face in the years ahead.

A regional map illustrating the location of RLWLH is shown in Figure 2.2.

Size. Rossmoor Leisure World, Laguna Hills occupies approximately 1,700 acres and has nearly 13,000 dwelling units. The population in 1981 was about 21,000.

History. The retirement community is the second Leisure World built by the Rossmoor Corporation. After the phenomenal success of the first Leisure World in Seal Beach, California, Ross Cortese,

---

[1]From an article in *Orange County Illustrated*, March 1979.

24

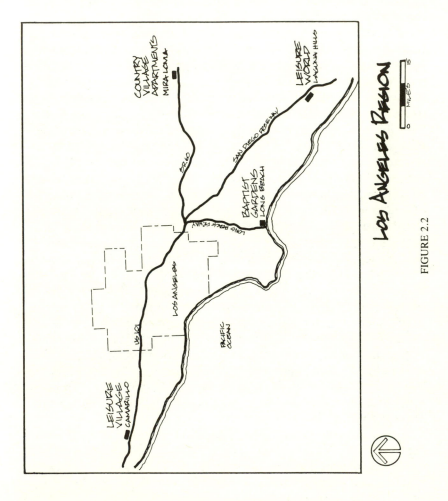

LOS ANGELES REGION

FIGURE 2.2

founder of Rossmoor, purchased more than 3,000 acres of the Moulton Ranch in the Saddleback Valley. The site was ideally located near the proposed San Diego freeway, but had no water or sewage disposal. To solve this problem Rossmoor tried to annex the property to Laguna Beach or Santa Ana. When these efforts failed, the company was forced to build its own facilities.

A more critical problem was posed by the opposition of the Marine Corps located at El Toro Marine Base to the north. They objected to the dense population that was planned below an approach path to the base. The El Toro Marines unit had been instructed by the Marine Corps Commandant in Washington, D.C. to vehemently oppose anything and everything which might affect the operation of the Marine Corps. In keeping with these orders, the Marines persuaded the County to deny approval of Rossmoor's application for zoning the property under the new planned community ordinance until Rossmoor agreed to certain restrictions on the use of the property. They also convinced FHA to revoke previously approved FHA insurance with the same requirement. In 1963 Rossmoor agreed to create a 500 acre green belt under the flight path. Use of this property is restricted to agriculture, recreation, and other low-density uses; housing is precluded. These restrictions forced Rossmoor to make major changes in the Master Plan of the RLWLH community.[2] With the restrictions imposed upon Rossmoor, the Marines withdrew their opposition and approval from the County for the zoning and FHA for the insurance were immediately given. Construction began and on September 10, 1964 the first residents moved to RLWLH.

FHA financing was the key to the Leisure World developments because it was so inexpensive that Rossmoor was able to provide extensive services and still keep prices low.[3]

Unfortunately, as mortgage rates shot up during the late 1960s, Rossmoor was forced to pay large discounts (the difference between the higher rates and the fixed FHA rates) in order to secure FHA financing. The company could not afford this and was forced to abandon the FHA program. It looked for a time as if RLWLH

---

[2]In 1967 Rossmoor brought suit against the Marines for compensation and was awarded $4.2 million in damages and interest. This, however, did not resolve all the problems, and in 1982 conflict over the use of the green belt area continues between Rossmoor and the Marines.

[3]Section 213, Title II of the National Housing Act allowed a 5¼ percent 40-year mortgage with only a 3 percent down payment.

would be completed at 6,000 units, one-third the originally planned size. Fortuitously, the State of California in 1968 adopted a uniform condominium law which gave Rossmoor an alternative. Since 1968 all housing in RLWLH has been sold as condominiums. Since then the development of RLWLH has progressed smoothly to its completion in 1981.

Philosophy

Rossmoor Leisure World was the creation of Ross Cortese, who wanted "to supply the basic needs of life for people aged 52 or older, create a serene atmosphere of beauty, provide recreation and religious facilities . . . then leave the living to the individual."

Resident Characteristics

Number of residents. The RLWLH population has grown steadily since the community opened in 1964, but not at the same rate. There was rapid growth during the first 5 years and then the growth slowed. Between 1965 and 1970, the population increased from 1,470 to 8,160. By 1975 the population had increased to 18,000, and by 1980 it had reached 21,000.

Admission requirements. Persons must be at least 52 years old to live in RLWLH. In the Towers the minimum age is 62. Prospective residents must also qualify financially, be free of a felony conviction for their entire lives and be free of a conviction for moral turpitude for 5 years.

Socioeconomic and demographic profile. Even though the average age of *new* residents has been decreasing since the mid-1970s, the average age of the entire RLWLH population has increased slightly since 1979, at which time the typical resident was 71 years old. In 1981, residents averaged 73 years old. Residents vary in age from 52 to over 100 and roughly half of the population is in the 70-79 year old age bracket.

The proportion of residents who are married couples has decreased since the community opened. About 80 percent of the initial residents were married and in 1981 about two-thirds were married. Additionally, 30 percent were single women and about 5 percent were single men. Most residents are white, Protestant, affluent, well-educated, and politically conservative. In the last few years the Jewish population has risen to about 10 percent.

Although most residents have middle and upper-middle class

backgrounds, there has been a continuous trend toward increasing affluence. When the community opened, persons with fixed incomes, either pensions or social security, were able to qualify financially; today many of these residents have difficulty meeting monthly payments. Nonetheless, the average net worth of the first residents, at the time they moved in, was $100,000; in 1981 the average net worth of new residents was considerably higher.

Nearly every occupation is represented in RLWLH, although the majority of residents are from professional occupations (doctors, lawyers, professors) or business (managers, executives). Early residents were predominantly blue collar or government workers, or teachers. In 1981, somewhat more than half of the residents had *at least* completed college and fewer than one in five have either some high school education or a high school degree.

Nearly all RLWLH residents are fully retired. About 10 percent continue in full-time careers and about 20 percent work part-time.

The more than 400 residents living in the Towers have similar backgrounds to the other RLWLH residents, but there are some differences. The average age is higher (82 versus 73), as is the average age of the purchaser (68 versus 64). The percentage of single women living in the Towers is also higher than for all of RLWLH. About 40 percent of Tower residents are married couples, 55 percent are single women and less than 10 percent are single men. Tower residents seem to be slightly more affluent too. The facility was designed as a luxury hotel and the extra services (see "Services and Facilities") increase the monthly carrying charges.

Residents of Rossmoor Leisure World, Laguna Hills are healthy and physically active, with a small proportion of the population having withdrawn from activity because of failing health. Some residents need personal assistance, but this is usually only temporary. RLWLH was designed for active adults, but there is no pressure to make residents leave if they are not ambulatory. While there are many active residents who are 80 years old and older, the number of residents needing some assistance is increasing as the population ages. To many residents and the staff, this is especially evident in the older sections of the community.

Residential history. Rossmoor Leisure World, Laguna Hills is the permanent home of nearly all its residents. There are a few seasonal residents and roughly a quarter of the population is traveling at any one time. Most residents move into RLWLH expecting to live there indefinitely and many do. Yearly turnover is only 5 percent.

About two-thirds of the residents lived in southern California before they moved into RLWLH and of these, about half came from within 2 hours of RLWLH. One-tenth of the population come from other parts of California and slightly more than one-fifth originate elsewhere, primarily from the midwest states.

Security is the primary reason people move into RLWLH, though until 1966 the medical services were the major attraction. However, passage of Medicare made this service less important. The recreation facilities, especially swimming pools and golf courses, also attract residents.

Residents leave RLWLH for a variety of reasons, e.g., they need more health care, to be near their families, because of the death of a spouse, or they are unable to meet community living expenses.

Level of activity. RLWLH residents are extremely active, placing a high demand on all the RLWLH facilities and programs. For the last 8 years swimming has been the most popular sport, and golf the second most popular sport. In the last few years residents' interest in physical fitness and exercise has increased. The result has been a burgeoning exercise program and a new mini-gym. Craft shops are also used extensively; about 15 percent of the residents enroll in various classes offered through the recreation department.

The breadth and variety of resident interests is evident in the nearly 200 clubs organized in RLWLH. There are professional clubs for academicians, dentists, lawyers, human concerns professionals; game clubs for enthusiasts of billiards, pinochle, and scrabble; sports clubs for every activity available in RLWLH and some, such as bowling, which are not; craft/art/hobby clubs for aficionados of photography, gardening, knitting, woodcarving; special interest clubs including a variety of dance and music clubs, as well as highly specialized interests like china dolls, petroleum, and Transcendental Meditation; and fraternal groups. Each club has a schedule of meetings, activities, and entertainment, including lectures, travel, and dinners, throughout the year. Nearly three-quarters of the residents belong to at least one club and many are so involved in club activities they have to carry an appointment book.

Many residents are also involved in helping to meet the changing needs of the population. For instance, a group was organized during the first years to help new residents get acquainted, especially single residents. Later, another group, the Institute for Living at Leisure World, was organized with much the same purpose, but focusing more on the needs of RLWLH friends as they grow old.

Few Towers residents use the community facilities. Instead they are active within the Towers, which has its own facilities and programs for the exclusive use of its residents. Popular activities for these residents are armchair exercises, bingo, cards, concerts, recitals, and movies.

Residents are also active outside RLWLH. All residents use the commercial and financial facilities in Laguna Hills. Residents are also politically active. Nearly 80 percent of them are registered to vote and voter turnout in RLWLH is 98%, twice that of other voters in the area. The RLWLH vote is usually conservative but residents have given continuous support to local education, including supporting bond issues.

Some residents take classes offered in the surrounding area. The RLWLH golfers, bowlers, and tennis players arrange tournaments with populations outside RLWLH, often with the residents of LW at Seal Beach. The RLWLH chess club also challenges local high school chess players to an annual competition.

Volunteer work is also a major activity and contribution of the residents. In 1980, for instance, volunteer activity at the hospital passed .5 million hours. Most of the time was contributed by the RLWLH volunteers; residents also volunteer their time and talents at the Thrift Shop which is operated to raise money for the hospital. They teach English as a second language, work with juveniles in the county boys' home, and counsel former drug addicts at the drug rehabilitation center. As part of their club activities residents also contribute money for scholarships, translate books into braille, and much more.

RLWLH residents and staff have excellent relations because of the precise definition of the duties and responsibilities of the staff as well as the "open-door" philosophy of the current management company.

This is not to imply that problems never occur. When they do it is usually the result of some change. For example, the lowered pool temperatures lasted only a few days once residents voiced their complaints.

Staff. In 1981 there were nearly 1,200 employees working for the management company of RLWLH in eight different divisions: general administration, community relations, financial services, personnel and security, recreation, Towers, maintenance, and landscaping. This is a staff-to-resident ratio of about 1-to-20. The company hires both full- and part-time help, union and non-union employees, skilled, semi-skilled, and unskilled labor. Personnel include the directors, and each Division's professional, office, and special staff. For example, the Recreation Division hires students doing field work, personnel with degrees in recreation and theatre, as well as residents who work as technicians, ushers, lifeguards, and starters at the golf course. Security includes armed, special deputies, resident security guards, and fire and safety marshals. Landscaping hires laborers (brushmen) and gardeners. The maintenance staff includes plumbers, electricians, janitors, and carpenters. Part-time employees include the 360 residents working as bus drivers, security guards, safety and fire marshals and in recreation as technicians, ushers, lifeguards, starters, and card attendants at the golf course. Full-time employees cannot live in RLWLH and most live within 25 miles.

Towers personnel include the manager, activities supervisor, building maintenance, housekeeping and meals service staff, and a nurse.

Overall staff turnover averages less than 2 percent a month but varies between divisions. Recreation staff has the lowest turnover, and landscaping the highest, due primarily to the seasonal help. Increased benefits in the last few years reduced turnover in key staff positions from nearly 40 percent a year to about 15 percent a year. Jobs in RLWLH are generally considered desirable because the pay is competitive and there is year-round employment.

Housing

Size and mix of housing stock. RLWLH contains approximately 13,000 dwelling units. Single-family detached dwellings, two to eight plexes and one-, two-, and three-story apartment buildings are arranged in clusters around open spaces. The Towers retirement residence is made up of two 14-story buildings containing 311 apartments.

The trend in RLWLH has been to upgrade the size and quality of housing. In response to market demand, smaller, mid-priced units have given way to larger and more expensive units. Nearly all units are two or three bedrooms, but some of the units built early in the development are one bedroom. The size of homes has increased over the years. The first units averaged 900 square feet; in the early 1970s units averaged 1,200 square feet, and by the late 1970s they were typically 1,600 square feet. The last units, sold in 1981, averaged 2,400 square feet.

There have been a variety of changes in the original plan for RLWLH in response both to financial changes in the housing industry and to demand. The original Master Plan proposed 18,000 units. These were to be cooperatively owned and built with FHA insured loans under Section 213. More than 6,000 units were built before 1968, when Rossmoor was forced to abandon the cooperative project and FHA financing in favor of condominium ownership. At this same time Rossmoor built the first three-story structure at RLWLH, called the Garden Villas. This building has 24 units and a recreation room with a kitchen and rest rooms.[4]

Single-family detached homes were built in 1972 for the first time. Since then, no more than 400 have been built because the low density made them too costly. Demand for the single-family homes, however, has not diminished.

Another major housing change was the building of the Towers. Plans for a new type of building with a broader range of services began in 1970. Rossmoor executives considered building a life-care facility, but feedback from residents indicated the desirability of congregate housing or a retirement residence.

In 1975 Rossmoor decided to abandon all prior building types and introduced a new architectural style because officials believed new sales had been competing with resales of the same design. Another change in housing occurred in building the last units of the project. Development of the final 533 units was about to begin when the company changed its plans, and decided to build 194 units of which 110 were large and luxurious homes. This decision was based on repeated requests from specific buyers.

Housing in specific geographic areas of RLWLH is owned by either a cooperative or a condominium corporation called a mutual. Each mutual owns all the common property within a designated area. In the cooperative form of ownership, the common property includes the land, buildings, and units. Residents are members of the mutual and own an equity share in it which gives them the right to occupy a particular unit. In condominium ownership the common property includes the land and buildings. Each resident holds title to a specific unit and is a member in the mutual which gives him/her ownership to an undivided share in the common property.

There are 85 mutuals in RLWLH ranging in size from 50 to 650

---

[4]Operation of this facility is the responsibility of building residents, not the RLWLH recreation department.

units. In 1967 these individual mutuals began to consolidate. By 1975 all 21 cooperative mutuals with over 6,000 units had formed the United Laguna Hills Mutual. In 1981 nearly all the condominium mutuals had consolidated into the Third Laguna Hills Mutual. The goal is for one cooperative corporation (United), a condominium corporation (Third Laguna), and the Towers.[5] Some mutuals have resisted consolidation. Mutual 14, for instance, is geographically isolated and a sense of separate identity developed among its residents for a period. Some of the final mutuals do not feel the pressure to consolidate that early mutuals did because there are now so few mutuals. The original argument for consolidation no longer holds, that is, that 85 mutuals is impossibly large.[6]

Costs to individuals. The sales price of new homes in RLWLH has increased over the years as homes have been upgraded in terms of size and quality and as inflation has acted on the local real estate market. Between 1964 and 1968, cooperative units sold from $12,000 to $24,000, or an average of $20 per square foot. In 1973 the price of homes ranged from $31,800 to $54,000, or an average of $35 per square foot. By 1977 prices had entered the $40,000 to $135,000 range, or an average of $55 per square foot, and the final units, sold in 1981, ranged in price from $320,000 to $350,000, or an average of $140 per square foot. This represents an overall increase of 600 percent over 17 years.

RLWLH real estate has also appreciated as evidenced by the data in Table 2.1.

Included in the purchase price of a unit is an initiation or membership fee to Golden Rain Foundation (GRF), the non-profit corporation which owns and operates the community property (see "Ownership/Governance/Management"). The fees collected from buyers are used to purchase or build facilities such as the golf courses and clubhouses. The fees have increased as costs have increased (see "Finance").

Residents also pay monthly carrying charges which cover the cost of operating the recreation, security, transportation, and other services; fees also pay for water; trash collection; cable TV; all exterior maintenance, repair, and upkeep; gardening and landscaping

---

[5]Cooperative and condominium mutuals cannot legally be consolidated. The Towers will never consolidate because of the greater variety of services offered.

[6]Mutuals are reluctant to consolidate for other reasons as well. They fear loss of identity, and like what is perceived as more personal attention from being small. Since 1980 a per unit surcharge has been levied for nonconsolidation.

Table 2.1

UNIT	1974 Unit Price	1976 Price/ % Increase	1977 Price/ % Increase	1980 Price/ % Increase
Coronado (coop)	$15,000	$19,500/30%	$28,000/45%	$42,000/50%
New Seville (coop)	$28,100	$33,000/20%	$53,100/60%	$75,000/40%
Coronado (condo)	$24,600	$25,800/5%	$34,700/35%	$54,000/55%
Villa Paraisa (condo)	$70,000	$95,000/35%	$146,700/55%	$200,000/40%

of common areas; street, sewer, and lighting maintenance; insurance administration fees; and certain medical services. The carrying charge in the cooperative mutuals, in addition, includes interior maintenance, replacement of appliances, mortgage, and taxes. In the condominium mutuals these are the responsibility of the individual owners.

The Towers monthly charges include the same services as any other condominium mutuals, plus paying for the meals, maid and janitorial, and medical services provided in the Towers.

Demand. RLWLH housing has always been in demand. The first 530 units, for instance, sold in an hour and a half and in 1977, 1,200 buyers competed for 240 homes. Since the mid-1970s Rossmoor has held drawings to determine buyers. Yearly sales volume, however, has dropped. In 1965 more than 2,000 units were sold and in 1967 more than 1,000 units were sold. Since 1968, however, yearly sales have averaged below 500 units. The periodic recessions in the national housing industry, for instance in the late 1960s and mid-1970s from increased mortgage rates, have also affected RLWLH sales. The problem, however, is not reduced demand but the difficulty of prospective purchasers to find buyers for their homes.

Demand for the Towers has not been as great as in the rest of the community. Enthusiasm for the Towers waned after it was built. It was expensive and came on the market in 1974, one of the worst sales years. The facility was also plagued by alleged construction problems, which led to a class action suit filed by the residents against Rossmoor. Tower units have not appreciated at the same rate as other units in RLWLH and in some cases the 1980 prices were actually lower than 1974 prices.

The problems with the Towers affected the entire RLWLH development since new construction depends upon new sales. Moreover, Rossmoor was committed to paying the monthly carrying charges on all unsold units, which was a financial drain on the company.

Facilities and Services (F/S)

F/S provided by Leisure World. Leisure World communities were conceived and designed to provide a particular life-style, new in the early 1960s, through extensive, planned services and facilities, for the exclusive use of residents. The emphasis was on recreation and leisure activities supported by security, transportation, landscaping, and maintenance services. More than any of the Leisure World communities, RLWLH embodies this dream.

Recreation facilities in RLWLH are diverse and grand. The six specialized clubhouses are the center for most recreation activities. Clubhouse I is the original facility. During the first years it housed all the management departments as well as a post office and bank. It has rooms for meetings, classes, dining, an art gallery, and a dark-room. It also has facilities for table tennis, billiards, lawn bowling, shuffleboard, badminton, and bocce ball, as well as swimming and hot pools. The most popular features are the recently built mini-gym and exercise room.

Clubhouse II has rooms for cards, meetings, lectures, and dining as well as facilities for billiards, lawn bowling, shuffleboard, tennis, and swimming.

Clubhouse III was designed and built by the RLWLH residents to be the entertainment center. It houses an auditorium/theatre which seats more than 800. It has rehearsal and dressing rooms, as well as rooms for dining, conferences, and billiards (non-smoking). It is the only clubhouse that does not have a swimming pool.

Clubhouse IV is the craft center with well-equipped studios for woodworking, sewing, lapidary, ceramics, slipcasting, photography, copper enameling, and jewelry making. Most studios also have classroom space. The clubhouse also has an art studio, multipurpose room, bridge rooms, and a swimming pool and hot pool.

Clubhouse V is the newest facility with large rooms for dining and lectures, conferences and classes. There are also rooms for billiards (non-smoking) and games. There is a hot pool and a solar heated swimming pool.

Clubhouse VI was originally built by Rossmoor for use by prospective buyers who wished to experience RLWLH life by spending 1 or 2 weeks in the community. It is the smallest clubhouse with only a small swimming pool as well as rooms for dining, parties and meetings, lounge areas, and a billiard room.

Also available to residents are extensive golf facilities including a 27-hole course and a 9-hole course, a driving range, putting greens, a pro-shop, and a practice area. Equestrian facilities include stables where residents can either rent or board horses and miles of trails. There are two garden centers with nearly 1,000 plots which residents rent on a yearly basis. Though not part of the original plan, they were quickly included when Cortese discovered the number of residents who wished to garden.

Another and unique facility is the Leisure World Library which started as a project for the Panhellenic Club. Through the efforts of club members and the support of the RLWLH community it has continued to grow and moved from a former game room in Clubhouse II into its own building in 1976. In 1981 the collection included 20,000 hardcover and 25,000 paperback books with a yearly circulation of 140,000.

These facilities are in high demand. Since 1975 annual usage has averaged 1.8 million person hours. Approximately three-quarters of this total is clubhouse use, which translates into about 600 person hours per clubhouse per day. The Recreation Division operates and maintains all these facilities. It is also responsible for assisting in the administration of clubs, coordinating classes offered either through the Emeritus Institute's staff or by other instructors and for scheduling clubhouse use. This Division plans and sponsors many of the events and activities while others are sponsored by the clubs. These activities include dances, dinners, theatre productions, lectures, movies, and much more.

Security is perhaps the most important RLWLH service, since it is the primary reason residents choose to live in the community. The security staff, composed primarily of residents, and headed by deputies from the Orange County Sheriff's Office, is primarily responsible for keeping unauthorized persons from entering the community. The guards man the 13 gates which give access into RLWLH through the brick walls topped by 2 feet of barbed wire. The wire was installed in 1976 for added security after a rash of petty thefts and much debate. Guards also patrol the community, inside and along the perimeter, 24 hours a day, 7 days a week. Security is also responsible for traffic and pet control and the coordination of emergency services, which includes responding to an emergency maintenance call after hours or assisting a resident who is locked out of his/her home. Though not entirely crime free, RLWLH has been cited by the Orange County Sheriff's Department as the safest area in the County.

RLWLH provides maintenance services for the entire community. These include sewer and water line repair and upkeep; routine plumbing, electrical, and carpentry maintenance; preventative work and major repairs such as painting of building exteriors and roof replacement; and the cleaning and repair of streets, sidewalks, and lighting. There is also a computerized service system which handles the calls from residents for maintenance service.

The Transportation Department, which is associated with the Maintenance Division, schedules and operates 18 minibuses. The buses run, free of charge, along 12 routes between the residential areas, clubhouses, stables, and garden centers and to nearby commercial and financial areas as well as the hospital. On a busy day ridership can reach 4,000 people. All 80 drivers are residents and trained in CPR. There is also a shuttle service to take residents home after scheduled evening events.

The Landscape Division is responsible for maintenance of 765 landscaped acres, including 50,000 trees and 800,000 shrubs. Residents may also call the service desk for assistance with particular landscaping problems.

All of these services are for the benefit and/or use of *all* RLWLH residents. Residents of the Towers, however, have additional services for their exclusive use. The Towers has its own recreation facilities and programs which are organized and run by the Towers recreation director and not through the Recreation Division. Recreation facilities include a 200-seat auditorium (the Great Hall) used for educational and recreational activities, lounges and card rooms, shuffleboard courts, two jacuzzi hot pools, and a Key Club. Programs offered include movies, lectures, parties, bingo, cards, concerts and recitals, special day and holiday events, and an armchair exercise program. Access to the building is restricted to Towers residents.

The Leisure World developments provide for the religious observance of residents. In Seal Beach, Rossmoor built a chapel within the community and planned to do the same at RLWLH. However, it became clear in the early years of development that RLWLH residents wanted to establish their own denomination churches. As a result, Cortese decided to offer land to each major religious group having a congregation of at least 100 RLWLH members. The only stipulation was that construction of a place of worship had to begin within 2 years. By 1968 seven churches and one synagogue had been built.[7] Most of the sites are along the perimeter of RLWLH and each church or temple is open to people living outside RLWLH.

F/S provided by governmental/philanthropic organizations. RLWLH is served by the Orange County Sheriff's Department and the California Highway Patrol. However, it is not patrolled by

---

[7]These houses of worship do not totally reflect the religious diversity of the residents, since many congregations continue to use clubhouse facilities for their services.

either force, since this is a private community. The California Department of Forestry, under contract to the Orange County Fire Department, also serves RLWLH. The station is adjacent to the community and was built on land sold by Rossmoor to the County and the first fire engine was a gift from Rossmoor.

A major service provided for RLWLH residents are the classes offered through the Emeritus Institute sponsored by the Saddleback Community College. RLWLH residents constitute one-quarter of all Emeritus Institute students. About 180 classes each year are conducted in the RLWLH clubhouses. The curriculum includes classes in physical fitness such as aerobic and strenuous conditioning, physical fitness, and folk dance; arts and crafts such as Chinese brush technique, watercolor, ceramics; and more academic subjects such as languages, estate planning, and stocks and bonds. The classes are open to anyone, but since they are only publicized within the RLWLH area non-residents have never exceeded 5 percent of the total enrollment.

Public transportation to nearby cities and airports is accessible at a shopping mall adjacent to RLWLH.

F/S provided by private enterprise. RLWLH opened development in the Saddleback Valley and attracted a variety of commercial, retail, professional, financial services and businesses. Many, such as the banks, savings and loans, and travel agencies, were drawn by the potential of serving primarily RLWLH residents. In 1976, amidst great controversy and some animosity, a mortuary was built immediately outside one of the RLWLH gates.

RLWLH residents have access to diverse communications media. Each dwelling is wired to a master antenna system. Channel 6 of this system is used for the community's closed circuit station. The station was originally operated by the Leisure World Foundation, the first management company of RLWLH (see "Management"). In 1968 a separate production company was formed which dissolved a year later but the station was kept going through the Recreation Division until its operation was taken over by Rossmoor Electric Inc.[8] in 1969. The programming is directed to the RLWLH residents and avoids duplication of what is available on other channels. Programs include game shows such as bingo and Fibber's Follies, cooking, travel, health and fitness shows, as well as Leisure World Today, a local news and interview program, and Trading Post,

---

[8]Rossmoor Electric is not part of or related to Rossmoor Corporation.

which is basically a classified ad service which also gives residents a chance to get acquainted. A program called "Administrative Chat" has been offered since the RLWLH opened and provides the management staff with the opportunity to discuss community issues, problems, questions, and changes. In recent years there has been an increased trend by mutual directors to take advantage of the communication opportunities of Channel 6.

The Leisure World News also began under the auspices of Leisure World Foundation. The newspaper serviced all Leisure World communities and was offered free of charge. It was sold when Leisure World Foundation was dissolved in 1972 and was taken over by Golden West Publishing Corp., a private enterprise. The paper carries the news of RLWLH, reporting on community issues and board and club meetings. It also carries ads from local and some national businesses. The offices are in the administrative building at RLWLH.

F/S provided by Leisure World for surrounding community. When the land for the RLWLH development was purchased in the early 1960s, approximately 1,300 acres were set aside by Rossmoor for commercial and other development. Rossmoor has been involved in most of this development, including five shopping malls, an office complex, age-integrated housing, a community for Christian Scientists, a plant nursery, and various other projects. It was the company's construction of Rossmoor Water Company and the Rossmoor Sanitation Company which made development in this area possible, not only for Rossmoor but other companies as well. Rossmoor also built roads which were later deeded to the County.

Some RLWLH residents have been active in the surrounding area. For instance, during the first years a group of residents built a motel (later sold) where their guests could stay. Residents also participate in various research projects conducted by universities, especially the University of California, and businesses such as Southern California Edison.

Facilities and services provided by RLWLH are summarized in Table 2.2.

Medical Care (MC)

MC provided by Leisure World. Ross Cortese envisioned the Leisure Worlds as communities providing all necessary services for the mature, including medical services. These services were modi-

Table 2.2

PROVIDERS OF FACILITIES AND SERVICES
(NON-MEDICAL)

Location	Retirement Community (Developer/Sponsor/Residents)		Governmental/ Philanthropic	Entrepreneurial
	RC Residents	Non-residents		
Inside RC	6 specialized clubhouses with rooms for crafts, games, meetings, classes, dining rooms, ballrooms, lounges, an art gallery, auditorium/theatre mini-gym library shuffleboard badminton bocce ball 5 swimming pools 5 hot tubs lawn bowling tennis 3 golf courses putting greens driving range pro-shop equestrian facilities garden plots activities program security maintenance transportation		classes	newspaper TV station
Outside RC		commercial churches water plant sewage plant volunteers	extensive cultural and recreation police & fire public transportation	commercial financial

40

fied in all Leisure Worlds with the passage of Medicare. In RLWLH other modifications resulted from financial pressures on Rossmoor. In RLWLH the original plan of medical services and facilities included a medical clinic, hospital, and complete medical insurance.[9]

The medical clinic was designed as the centerpiece of the medical program. The facility was built by Rossmoor and leased by the Golden Rain Foundation (GRF) which purchased both the clinic and adjacent land in 1968. Until 1972, when GRF sold it to the hospital, the clinic provided office space for private doctors, including specialists in surgery, neurology, dermatology, and orthopedics, available by appointment to residents. The clinic also had a pharmacy, lab facilities, x-ray, and ambulance services. The clinic nursing staff assisted the doctors in office appointments and made home visits through the most valuable service, the Home Care Program. This service provided home nursing care as ordered by a doctor, as well as 24-hour doctor-nurse emergency service. Medicare, passed in 1966, required the clinic to establish a Home Health Agency for certification. This program incorporated and expanded on the former Home Care Program. It included a variety of rehabilitation services including physical and speech therapy as part of the home care and the services of a social worker.

The passage of Medicare also eliminated the need for the medical insurance program which had provided 80 percent coverage for in- and out-patient medical care and medication.[10] These costs were paid through the monthly carrying charges and the remaining 20 percent was billed to the patient.[11]

Rossmoor originally planned to build the hospital in 1965, adjacent to the medical clinic. Construction was about to begin when the company announced it was unable to finance the construction and requested that it be released from further responsibility. This was unpleasant news for RLWLH residents. The medical services were the primary reasons residents moved to RLWLH and the advertising for the community featured the hospital. Moreover, with 2,000

---

[9]In Seal Beach and Maryland, only a clinic and medical insurance were planned. A hospital, however, was part of the plan for the Walnut Creek Leisure World.

[10]The decision to eliminate the RLWLH program was not easy, however, since it provided coverage for all residents and Medicare is only for persons 65 and older. The administration never found a satisfactory means for continuing the RLWLH program for younger residents.

[11]The medical program in LW Seal Beach started with 100 percent coverage, but resident abuse was so costly the program had to be changed to 80-20 coverage.

elderly residents, a hospital close to the community was needed. GRF began to explore alternatives and eventually assumed responsibility for construction. The major obstacle to construction of any hospital was financing. GRF did eventually secure a Hill-Burton grant and donated $800,000. The funds for this donation were obtained by increasing the initial membership fee from $500 to $1,200 in 1966.

Golden Rain Foundation (GRF) first considered building the hospital for the sole use of RLWLH residents, but was advised that this would be economically unfeasible. Eventually they built a non-profit hospital to serve the entire Saddleback Valley. A separate corporation was formed to sponsor the hospital and construction began in 1971. In 1972, GRF decided to sell the medical clinic to the hospital thereby avoiding duplication of services such as the lab and pharmacy. The clinic then became the out-patient medical clinic for the entire hospital. Saddleback Valley Community Hospital opened in 1974. RLWLH residents continue to control the hospital board and constitute the majority of patients and volunteer staff.

When GRF sold the clinic to the hospital, it arranged to contract for the continuation of 24-hour emergency home care, as had been available through the clinic. Recently, however, this service has become controversial. Some residents question the need for home visits by a doctor and nurse and see it only as a RLWLH hospital subsidy. In fact, extensive ambulance and paramedic services have reduced the need for this service since ambulance services are willing to respond to calls for personal assistance, such as helping a resident back into bed, in exchange for exclusive rights of access of RLWLH.

Residents also have a variety of health related services and facilities available to them within the community. Both homemaker services, introduced in 1966, and social workers are available through the Human Relations Department of the Community Relations Division. The former coordinates resident hiring of homemakers and practical nurses who assist ill or infirm residents in their homes. The social worker or human relations services provide counseling, information, and referral services. The need and demand for this service has grown as the community has grown and as the service's reputation has been established. When the community was young the primary responsibility of the social worker was to check on people; counseling was short-term. Today there are more acute, long-term, crises intervention cases. One of the major issues is second retirement, i.e., retirement from active life, and time is spent counseling residents on how to plan for or adapt to a less active life-style or a possible move to a continuing care facility.

Security guards respond to emergency medical calls within RLWLH, often arriving before the paramedics. At least two guards, trained in CPR and first aid, are on duty at all times.

Also available for residents is the drop-in lounge, organized in 1981 by the Institute for Living, a RLWLH club. The lounge has been valuable in attracting residents who had withdrawn from activities and helps to get them involved again. It provides social refreshment along with the coffee served to anyone who wants to drop in. It is run entirely by volunteers. In Clubhouse V there is the Friendship Center, operated by the Human Relations Division. It provides a meeting place for residents for friendly conversation and counseling. It is staffed by specially trained volunteers. To meet the very difficult need for transportation the Human Relations Department keeps names of resident volunteer drivers.

Towers residents have access to these services as well as additional ones for their exclusive use. It has a small clinic with an examination room and bed and equipment for resident use such as walkers, wheelchairs, and oxygen. A nurse is on-call within the Towers 24 hours a day. There is also an emergency call system between the residents' apartments and the nurse's clinic. The Towers also arranges for homemaker services for its residents.

In recent years there has been growing concern among residents that an increasing number of their friends have moved from RLWLH because they needed more health care than what was available in the community. Since no continuing care facilities exist in the immediate area, residents are forced to move away. This has been emotionally disruptive for all parties affected and provided the impetus for considering building such a continuing care facility for RLWLH residents.

Within the community there is an 18 acre site which could be used for such a facility, and financing could be secured. However, not all residents support the idea and some fear building a continuing care retirement center will blur the image of RLWLH and reduce property values.

MC provided by governmental/philanthropic organizations. Orange County has an extensive range of social and health services.

For instance, there is a crisis intervention center and elder care which offers counseling, checks blood pressure and vision, and performs glaucoma screening. The County runs a hospice, a mental health clinic, and a visiting nurse service, as well as dial-a-ride and dial-a-lift. The paramedics are part of the fire station.

Saddleback Community Hospital, adjacent to RLWLH, also has special services for the elderly as well as regular hospital services. The former include a discharge nurse to arrange for follow-up care, meals-on-wheels, an adult day-health care center with a program of therapy, counseling, nursing care, therapeutic assistance, recreational and social activities, nutritional counseling, and a mid-day meal. The hospital continues to operate the home health agency.

The Saddleback Community College conducts a popular and extensive exercise and fitness program for RLWLH residents. It offers supervised exercise based on evaluation of individual needs. There are special swimming programs and classes for the handicapped.

The Saddleback Kiwanis also offer free blood pressure screenings in RLWLH for residents.

MC provided by private enterprise. Laguna Hills has numerous private doctors, as well as ambulance service, nurse registries, meal services, and small group homes with either hotel service or custodial care. The latter especially have been drawn by the RLWLH population and are usually for temporary care only. In the immediate area there is only one convalescent hospital, Beverly Manor, which was built after RLWLH opened. Its presence was encouraged by GRF in the late 1960s when the need for a hospital was first recognized. Beverly Manor opened in 1968 next to the medical clinic on land owned by GRF.

MC provided by Leisure World for the surrounding area. It was through the efforts of RLWLH residents that Saddleback Community Hospital was built to serve the entire Saddleback community. RLWLH residents also encouraged the building of Beverly Manor.

RLWLH residents also run a thrift shop which sells resident-donated clothes. It makes about $120,000 a year which is donated to the hospital. It is run by volunteers, mostly from RLWLH, as is the hospital gift shop which also provides income for the hospital, about $12,000 a year.

Residents have also participated in various medical studies such as the University of Southern California exercise program.

Medical facilities and services provided by RLWLH are summarized in Table 2.3.

Table 2.3

PROVIDERS OF MEDICAL CARE

Location	Retirement Community (Developer/Sponsor/Residents)		Other Providers (Govt./Philanthropies/Private)
	RC Residents	Non-residents	
Inside RC	social services homemaker services Towers: emergency nursing		
Outside RC	hospital medical clinic	hospital medical clinic	convalescent hospital doctors county services ambulance home nursing homemaker care-homes paramedic 24-hour emergency service day-care

Ownership/Management/Governance

Type of ownership. RLWLH was developed by Rossmoor Corporation of California on land purchased in 1962. All housing is owned by individual, non-profit mutual corporations or homeowners associations. All community property and facilities such as the clubhouses, golf courses, and so on are owned by the Golden Rain Foundation, a non-profit corporation which holds these properties in trust for the benefit and use of the RLWLH residents.

Type of management/governance. Governance is an integral part of both cooperative and condominium forms of ownership and thus the community is governed by the several mutual corporations and the Golden Rain Foundation. Each corporation has the responsibility for operating and maintaining the grounds and buildings it owns. The duties of the mutual corporations are discharged by a Board of Directors elected by the residents of the mutual. The duties of all the mutual boards are virtually the same. They establish monthly carrying charges and rules pertaining to the rights and obligations of the residents and the use of the common area; they approve the budget[12] and set policy for the mutuals which can be as detailed as the painting schedule of the buildings. In cooperative mutuals the board also has the responsibility for accepting and rejecting membership applications of prospective residents.

The Golden Rain Foundation is responsible for operating and maintaining the community property and facilities and for providing various services such as transportation, security, and recreation. It also establishes rules for the use of community property including traffic regulations, pet control, pool hours, and so on. These responsibilities are discharged by a Board of Directors composed of 15 members serving 3-year staggered terms.[13] GRF directors are elected by the directors of the mutual boards with votes weighted by the number of units in the mutual.

The Golden Rain Foundation was first organized in 1960 in the first Leisure World Community at Seal Beach. It was created as an FHA requirement for the purpose of holding community property and facilities in trust for the residents and to provide certain ser-

---

[12]FHA has final authority over the budget, monthly carrying charges, and plan of operations for all cooperative mutuals.

[13]In 1972 GRF changed its by-laws to limit the number of directors to 15. Prior to this, GRF directors were chosen from each mutual board. As the community grew, so did the number of directors, approaching an unwieldy number and creating the need for change.

vices. GRF is not the umbrella corporation of the RLWLH community though this is a common misconception. It has control only over the property it owns and thus shares an equal responsibility for the community with the mutual corporations. This is a change from the original governance organization established in the Seal Beach Leisure World. In that community GRF is the ultimate authority and this created problems, such as an excess of power over all the residents being held in the hands of a few residents. It also diminished the power of the mutual corporations over their own property which led to conflict. These problems have been avoided in RLWLH because of the balance of power achieved through the change in organization.

Each mutual corporation and GRF sign a management contract with the same management company to perform certain tasks for them. These include hiring employees, contracting for services, purchasing supplies and equipment, collecting monthly carrying charges, keeping insurance, books, and records, and preparing a budget with a plan of operation. It is the responsibility of the management company to advise all the governing boards and to act in accordance with the policy set by each board.

The first management company of RLWLH was the Leisure World Foundation (LWF), a non-profit California corporation, formed in 1962 as an FHA requirement for the purpose of sponsoring, managing, and selling the Leisure World developments. FHA imposed this requirement as protection against failure of the community through weak and/or inadequate management. When Rossmoor switched to condominiums in 1968 the LWF was no longer necessary and by the early 1970s all Leisure World communities, except RLWLH, had terminated their LWF contracts. At this time the residents of RLWLH, concerned with the trademark implications of LWF, were considering finding a new management company. The LWF executives also wanted to form a for-profit management company and in 1972, Professional Management Company (PMC) was formed, retaining the LWF personnel and assuming management responsibility of RLWLH in January 1973. As of 1981, PMC continues to serve the RLWLH community.

As the RLWLH community evolved, changes occurred in the organization, the role of the governing corporations, and in the management company. The two most significant changes were the consolidation of the mutuals and the shift of power with increasing resident control.

The growing number of mutuals were increasing administrative costs and threatening to make administration impossible by virtue of their number. This became the impetus for consolidation in 1967 (see "Housing").

The shift in power to increasing resident involvement and control in governance occurred between 1973 and 1976. Until that time primary leadership was assumed by the management staff of the Leisure World Foundation. There were several reasons for this. For one thing, the concept of cooperative living was new and a process to be simultaneously learned and created by both management and residents. The management staff, however, had experience from work in Seal Beach, whereas many residents did not realize or anticipate their responsibility in governance when they entered RLWLH. Of all the corporations involved in running RLWLH (mutual, GRF, and management), only management was responsible for the entire community and was thus a unifying force. Also, during the first decade, the management staff remained relatively unchanged whereas the rapid and continuous growth of the community meant the formation of new boards and new directors who had to learn the operation of the community. It was natural for management to assume the role of educator.

After the first decade, however, many of these factors were no longer pertinent. By 1973 the population was 16,000 or three-fourths of its ultimate size. Growth slowed considerably about 1974 due to the depressed housing industry. Additionally, the number of residents experienced in running the community had increased. In essence, residents were ready to assume greater control of their community.[14] The charge of paternalism on the part of management, which residents had expressed over the years, was voiced more loudly indicating the changes in residents' expectations.

As resident involvement increased from 1973 to 1976, there was a clash with management. Residents began to question the competence and interests of PMC. Specifically, the PMC President was accused of lack of leadership and perceived as having a conflict of interest between his RLWLH obligations and other business interests.[15] These allegations led to a request for an outside evaluation of

---

[14]This readiness was heralded in 1972 when GRF revised its by-laws to prohibit the Administrator from serving as GRF President, as had been the case for the previous 6 years.

[15]When LWF was dissolved a separate corporation was formed to assume responsibility for publishing the Leisure World News. The LWF-PMC President held a controlling interest in this corporation and in the company which did data processing for PMC, raising charges of conflict of interest.

PMC, its operations, and personnel in 1976. The results were reassuring. PMC was found to be doing an excellent job. The only criticism was in the organizational structure which, the evaluation concluded, permitted inadequate leadership. Organizational changes were subsequently made to correct this. This included some staff changes; it was painful to some residents to see friends leave. The overall result was to help settle the issue of the locus of control. The community since then has been run with a clear understanding that GRF and the mutual boards set firm policies which management carries out. In other words, "The difference between 'the responsibility to advise' and the 'authority to decide' is very clear."[16]

Future changes in governance may occur if RLWLH residents decide to incorporate. This would create a new layer of government and, according to the general manager, require overall community leadership which would probably be assumed by GRF. It would also politicize the community. However, according to a former GRF President, it is not likely that residents would run for city office.

Degree of resident involvement in governance. The RLWLH community is run by its residents. All the directors of the various boards are residents as are the members of the various committees which provide policy advice and counsel to the mutual boards, GRF, and PMC. However, only one-fifth of the residents are actually involved in governance. The remainder are involved in enjoying it.

There are always people, in a community of this size, who want to lead. Others are drawn into leadership positions from a need to be reassured about the way things are being run. According to one staff member, many residents have to learn to trust management, especially to be able to write a check and give control for spending it to someone else. Their involvement as directors allays these fears.

On the whole, RLWLH residents are protective of their community and any threat to their way of life stimulates involvement. Change typically will generate activity and, during periods of change, RLWLH has experienced intense resident involvement, through informal structures. For instance, at the time of conversion to condominiums, two groups were formed—the Fact Finders and Club 16. Each was suspicious of management and questioned everything that happened. The Fact Finders eventually ran out of issues and dissolved; Club 16 continues to exist to keep its members informed.

---

[16]Taken from the materials provided for new board members by PMC.

In 1976, during the period of transition, the Community Association emerged. Their primary concern at the time was the secrecy with which they saw the community being run. Their claims were not entirely unfounded. According to one member of the management staff, things were not being fully explained because of the changes management was making. The Community Association's major concern was with the GRF and mutual boards, which, they claimed, were also operating in secrecy and making decisions behind closed doors. Again, their claims were not unjustified and their challenge contributed to the institution of open meetings. Today the Community Association continues as a forum for information exchange. The president has identified issues which will probably be rallying points in the future, including Rossmoor's proposed development of the green space, incorporation, and increasing fees.

Both the Fact Finders and the Community Association have been characterized as militant and critical, assuming crookedness and deceit exist. This perception undermines their constructive role and they easily become targets of anger and ridicule. Yet, the formation and activity of these groups seems only to be a different manifestation of the shift to greater resident involvement and the process of learning about cooperative living, which requires that mutual trust be established. RLWLH residents were described in the PMC evaluation as "articulate, forceful, involved and result-oriented (with) high expectations of service levels." This is evident in all forms of resident involvement and, whereas it does not always lend itself to peace and harmony, it does insure a dynamic and viable community.

Financing

Initial costs. Prior to the sale of the first home, Rossmoor had invested $15 million in the RLWLH development. These costs covered the purchase of the land ($2,300-$2,800/acre), building Clubhouse 1 (more than $1 million), an 18-hole golf course (more than $2 million,) and the sales pavilion, models, water and sewage treatment plants, streets, and so on. The President of Rossmoor estimates that 1981 costs for the same initial development would reach $150 million.

The investment in housing was also substantial. According to a 1968 Los Angeles Times story, FHA had approved $100 million in loans and residents had invested over $120 million in down payments.

Operating costs. There are three categories of operating expenses: direct mutual operating (DMO), mutual shared operating (MSO), and GRF shared operating. Direct mutual expenses include electricity, water, and sewage for each mutual. These costs vary between each mutual and are divided among the number of units in the mutual. Mutual shared and GRF shared expenses include administrative and maintenance services. These are divided equally between all the units. There are also other expenses including reserve funds for GRF and all the mutuals, and, in the cooperative mutuals, taxes, insurance, and mortgage principal and interest.

Expenses in the community have increased primarily with inflation, though management has successfully kept the increases below the inflation rate of Orange County. Between 1971 and 1980, for example, the shared expenses increased from $60/unit/month to $130/unit/month. Nearly two-thirds of this increase occurred after 1977, mostly due to increases in petroleum products.

Increasing costs are probably the major concern of residents. There are some who would like to end the shared concept and change to separate charges for services. The reasoning behind this position is the differential maintenance costs between mutuals, which, it is argued, impose an unfair burden on some mutuals. The financial services director of RLWLH, however, argues for the shared concept, stating that in fact it keeps costs down and has a psychological benefit for residents, since they know they can use anything without considering the cost. The shared concept also helps keep down fees that are charged for use, such as for the golf course. In 1981 a round of golf cost $3 and the financial services director estimates this would *at least* double if the shared concept were abandoned and everything were charged on a fee-for-service basis.

PMC has also found an effective way to keep down administrative expenses. It owns and operates the PMC-Resale Office, which handles about 80 percent of the yearly resales. Profits from these sales are used to defray administrative costs.

Tax structure. Property taxes for GRF property are included in the monthly carrying charges of the units. Residents of United Laguna, the cooperative mutual, also pay taxes as part of their carrying charges, whereas residents of condominium mutuals pay taxes on their own unit. Both the tax rate and the assessed land value have increased over the years. For example, the land which Rossmoor purchased in 1962 for $2,300 an acre was worth about $250,000 an acre in 1981.

Proposition 13 has had significant impact on unincorporated areas such as Laguna Hills. The restrictions it imposes on increasing taxes has reduced revenues, which has subsequently cut into services. It has become necessary to either cut services or provide them on a fee basis. Demand, however, has not diminished. As these changes occur in the Laguna Hills area there will be an increasing move toward incorporation which will provide a broader, stable tax base for the incorporated area, rather than having to depend on the allocation of funds from the County. A more immediate impact of Proposition 13 was the elimination of the adult education programs administered through the high school. This eliminated at least 30 classes that had been offered to RLWLH residents.

Sources of revenue. Monthly carrying charges are the primary source of revenue and are set to cover the operating costs of the entire community. They increase as costs increase.

There are two major sources of income for the RLWLH community—monthly carrying charges and the GRF membership fee, both paid by residents. The membership fee is included in the purchase price of the housing units. It is the primary source of revenue for construction of new facilities. It has increased as construction costs have increased and as the needs of the community have changed. For instance, when RLWLH opened, the fee was $450; the fee was increased in 1966 from $500 to $1,200 to collect money for the purchase of the medical center and construction of the hospital. By 1972 the fee was $1,825, in 1973 it had increased to $2,575, and by 1979 it was $4,300. There is also a "transfer fee" which is included in the price of resales. In 1968 it was set at $240, by 1978 it had increased to $1,750 and in 1979 it was $2,600.

Monthly carrying charges are based on the actual operating expenses of the entire community and increase as costs increase. They have not increased greatly as the costs have been kept down. For instance, in the cooperative mutuals between 1971 and 1980, income from cooperative mutuals increased only about 40 percent.

There are other sources of revenue, such as interest income, but these constitute less than 5 percent of the total cooperative income. GRF also charges various fees to defray costs of operating certain facilities and to curtail demand. Fees, for instance, are charged for resident use of the golf course and stables, as well as guest use of the pools and golf course, and so on.

Marketing and Plans for the Future

Advertising. In the late 1950s Ross Cortese identified what he believed was a neglected market, mature adults faced with rising property taxes, decaying municipal services, threatened personal safety, and changing neighborhoods. Moreover, he recognized the trend toward early retirement, increasing social security benefits and greater personal family savings, better pension plans, longer life spans, and increasing desire to get more out of retirement, all of which made the market desirable from a developer's viewpoint. He concluded this group needed more than just housing and created a new, totally planned community which offered shelter and an extensive package of services. In the early 1960s, the Rossmoor corporation began to build Leisure World communities.

Rossmoor was restricted by the FHA from any involvement in marketing these communities. This became the responsibility of the Leisure World Foundation until the conversion to condominiums, at which time Rossmoor was free to take over the marketing. The demand for homes in RLWLH was great during the first few years, in part because of the limited supply of housing in California. During this period it was more a problem of trying to keep up with demand than to create it.

The situation changed in the late 1960s and then again in the early 1970s as Rossmoor, along with the entire housing industry, was confronted with a depressed market brought about by increasing interest rates. This led the company to reexamine its marketing strategy. They discovered that the common perception of RLWLH was as an old folks home. This prompted a change in their approach so as to put greater emphasis on the selling of a life-style.

Rossmoor has used all types of media for advertising, including newspapers (local, Los Angeles Times), radio, magazine ads, and direct mail solicitation. Nearly three-quarters of all buyers have seen a newspaper ad for RLWLH, but 60 percent said they became interested in making a purchase after hearing about the community from friends or relatives.

With the completion of RLWLH Rossmoor's involvement will end and advertising will fall to individual real estate offices including PMC-Resales. Since three-quarters of all resales are the result of referrals from residents, the key element in any program is satisfied residents, and this is largely the responsibility of the management company. PMC-Resales has concluded there is no need to advertise nationally; they have, however, designed a color brochure for limited distribution and are working with the savings and loans and newspapers. PMC-Resales plans to give the papers stories about RLWLH, assuming that good stories will spread.

Future plans. The development of RLWLH was completed in 1981 and Rossmoor's involvement with the community, after 20 years, officially ended. In June 1981, the stockholders voted to liquidate the company. Some decisions remain, however. A major concern is the disposition of 170 acres of undeveloped property which are part of the green belt under the flight path of the Marine Corps. Rossmoor wants to sell the site for development as a business office park, but federal restrictions prevent this.

With the end of Rossmoor's involvement, the future of RLWLH is entirely in the hands of the residents. They face the new and challenging issues of a completed rather than a growing community.

Overview—Impacts of Change

Effects of change in Leisure World. During its nearly 20-year history RLWLH has experienced many changes, especially in its population. There has been a trend toward younger, more affluent residents, most noticeably since 1977. These residents have brought a different, more athletic life-style and new expectations about governance, recreation, and so on. In the GRF Five Year Capital Improvement Plan, a generation gap was identified. These differences could impact on the operation and maintenance of the Recreation Division by creating new demands. It is also feared that these differences, particularly as they exist among the residents of the final 110 units, could create cliquishness and there have been distressing rumors of the formation of the 110 Club.

The average age of the residents has been increasing and, in 1981, it was unclear if it would stabilize (at about 75 years old) or if it would continue to increase. In any event, there are already increasing demands on the RLWLH social services and need for greater health care. The latter has been the major reason for considering construction of a continuing care facility and the establishment of a standing health care committee.

In 1981 a major turnover in governance was beginning as directors, who had served the maximum 12-15 years on committees and various boards, were being replaced. According to the general manager, this break in continuity will be disruptive to the communi-

ty and will require education and training of new directors. Moreover, in the last few years residents have been reluctant to serve.
The community also faces an increasing need for overall leadership,
especially as the incorporation issue is examined. GRF is the most
likely candidate to assume this role.

Increasing costs is the biggest problem RLWLH confronts, now
and in the future. Though management has successfully kept expense increases below the inflation rate through cost-cutting measures, these measures are limited. As costs increase it is going to be
increasingly difficult to meet resident demand for quality services.
This may eventually lead to abandonment of the shared cost concept
in favor of fee-for-service. The situation is made worse by such
things as the increasing difficulty in getting residents to fill staff
positions in security and transportation. Costs will increase dramatically if it becomes necessary to hire outside staff. Already, increased fees have affected some residents, especially in the cooperative units. It can be expected that more will continue to have trouble
making it.

RLWLH is a powerful force within the Saddleback Valley. The
community opened development in the area and began the transfor-
mation from ranch land to urban area. The major consequences of
the subsequent, rapid growth have been intensified traffic and crime
problems. Other consequences have been positive. RLWLH attracted all types of development and, according to various county
officials, established a standard of quality which has influenced all
other development.

The concentration of elderly population has attracted various
businesses and services, such as travel agencies, financial planners,
savings and loans, and doctors specializing in geriatric medicine. To
compete for the RLWLH resident dollar, businesses also offer
special services. Restaurants, for instance, have early bird specials,
savings and loans and banks offer free coffee and traveler's checks.
RLWLH has also increased the awareness of the needs of the elderly
among county officials and citizens generally.

RLWLH residents are politically powerful and some people believe election to any office in the Saddleback Valley is impossible
without their vote. Their impact has been particularly evident in the
educational domain. In their continual support of education,
RLWLH residents have reflected their belief in its importance. In
the early days, when RLWLH represented the major population of
the Saddleback Valley, it was their vote which financed the forma-

tion of the new Saddleback Valley School District. Moreover, it is not possible to get elected to the school board without RLWLH backing. The community has affected education in other ways as well. For instance, the Saddleback Valley Community College was the first in the State to offer an associate of arts degree in gerontology.

RLWLH has been an attractive community for the County. It generates a sizable tax revenue and has minimal service requirements. The County does not have to build schools, provide public maintenance of streets, lighting, and landscaping, or provide water and sewage services. RLWLH does generate a higher demand on paramedic services, but a disproportionately low demand on fire and police services.

Effects of change in the surrounding community. Changes in the surrounding area have had fewer impacts on RLWLH. The community is affected by the increasing traffic problems and the increasing crime problems. As the surrounding area continues to grow, the political power of RLWLH is diminished. This is a partial impetus for considering incorporation, which would increase the RLWLH voice. Another concern is to protect against being included in someone else's incorporation plan by incorporating first.

RLWLH is a private community with an anti-solicitation policy. The community reserves the right to restrict outsiders from entering. This right has been challenged in a court case which may end up in the Supreme Court. Suit was brought by the News Post, a Laguna Beach newspaper which was denied access to deliver free newspapers to residents.

Summary

Rossmoor Leisure World, California is a "retirement new town." It is one of several Leisure World communities built by Rossmoor Corporation. Its evolution has been shaped by the continuous adaptation of the developer, residents, and management to changing conditions and problems.

A major problem for Rossmoor was the periodic depressions in the housing industry. High mortgage interest rates reduced sales and prolonged development. The most severe impact occurred in the late 1960s. Increasing interest rates forced Rossmoor to abandon the Section 213 program. Instead, the company introduced condominium ownership.

Rossmoor has responded to market changes by building larger, more expensive homes. As a result of this trend, younger, more affluent residents have moved into RLWLH. They, in turn, brought a different life-style and expectations. Rossmoor has also been responsive to resident demands. Their suggestions led to construction of the Towers and new recreational facilities.

Development of RLWLH was unique among the Leisure World communities because of Ross Cortese's personal involvement. The elegance and grand scale of this community reflect his imprint.

Residents and management have worked together to adapt the community to the changing needs, problems, and interests of the residents. In the late 1960s the residents built a hospital to meet immediate health needs. Management modified and expanded its social service program to meet the changing social and emotional needs of residents as they age. Residents have organized clubs and facilities, especially for single residents. Most recently, declining health of aging residents stimulated interest in providing more extensive medical care. Residents are considering building a continuing care center within RLWLH.

Management responded to the developing threat of crime by increasing security. When interest in exercise increased, residents responded by building a mini-gym and expanding the exercise program to accommodate residents of all levels of physical ability. These are only a few examples of how this community, through expansion, addition, and modification of services, has accommodated to change.

Governance has evolved as RLWLH has grown and as residents have learned about its operations. This evolution has been punctuated by changes in leadership. In about 1972 residents began to push for more control and management's power waned. This was coupled with a period of disruption which led to a reorganization of the administrative structure and redefinition of the roles of management and the various resident boards. In 1981 another period of change was beginning as the old guard retired from board positions and new leaders emerged. The future is likely to bring further change. GRF may assume the role of central leadership in the community, especially as the issue of incorporation is resolved. Resident involvement will probably lessen because of increasing reluctance of residents to serve on boards.

The most persistent problem has been increasing costs. Management instituted a highly successful cost-cutting program including energy conservation and an experimental program with plant growth. They have also imposed user fees on some recreational facilities. Many residents want to abandon the shared expense concept in favor of a fee-for-service arrangement. Cost reduction has also been achieved through consolidation of the mutuals.

SUN CITY,[17]
ARIZONA

General Description

Sun City, Arizona is a completely self-contained and unincorporated retirement "new town" composed of conventionally built residential structures and other land uses. It contains a complete assortment of facilities one would expect in any community: shopping centers, recreation facilities, churches, a hospital, medical clinics, gas stations, and restaurants. Although the for-profit developer, Del E. Webb Development Company (DEVCO), did not provide any medical or nursing facilities, they have been provided within Sun City by various independent groups. In order to live in Sun City, at least one member of the household must be 50 or more years of age.

Sun City was founded in 1960 and promoted as an "active retirement community." Since it has been such an enormous success, it has been called the "standard of the world in resort-retirement living." A site plan of Sun City is provided in Figure 2.3.

Location. Sun City is located 12 miles northwest of Phoenix, Arizona, in Maricopa County. For the most part, there are irrigated farms to the east and south of Sun City and desert areas to the north and west. The average maximum and minimum temperatures there are about 86 degrees and 52 degrees, respectively. Precipitation totals for the area average about 7.5 inches per year.

The 1970s were a period of rapid growth for Arizona and the Phoenix area. Between 1970 and 1979, Arizona's population grew by one million, an increase of 52 percent, representing the highest rate of growth on record for the State. Fifty-five percent of Arizona's total population lives in Maricopa County. Maricopa

---

[17]Much of the information reported in this case study was taken from the following: *This is Sun City* by the League of Women Voters, Sun City, Arizona, 1979; *Foresight Eighty* by the Western Savings and Loan Association of Phoenix, Arizona, 1980; and numerous documents provided by the Del E. Webb Development Company.

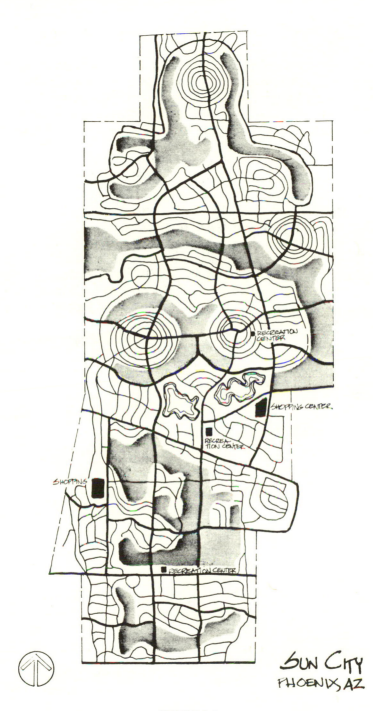

RECREATION
CENTER

SHOPPING CENTER.

RECREA-
TION CENTER

SHOPPING

RECREATION CENTER

SUN CITY
PHOENIX AZ

FIGURE 2.3

59

County's 1980 population was about 1.5 million, with more than half of the residents living in Phoenix. The Phoenix area is expected to increase by 14 percent in the 1980s to a population of 900,000 by 1990.

A regional map illustrating the location of Sun City is contained in Figure 2.4.

Size. In 1981, Sun City had a population of 47,600 people occupying 25,500 dwelling units. With this population, Sun City ranks as the seventh largest city in Arizona. The community contains 8,900 acres of land, or 14 square miles. The land on which Sun City was built is seven miles long in the north-south direction and about two and a half miles wide at its widest point.

History. Sun City was the idea of the late Del E. Webb, a Phoenix carpenter who built a multi-million dollar corporation. He envisioned a community where people over 50 years of age could lead active and leisurely lives in a pleasant climate. Sun City was to become the first of its kind: a new town for retirement.

The land on which Sun City was built (8,900 acres) was owned by

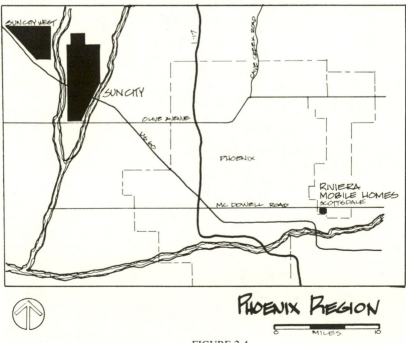

FIGURE 2.4

the J. G. Boswell Company and used to grow cotton and lettuce. In 1960, Webb joined with Boswell and formed the Del E. Webb Development Company to develop Sun City. Boswell owned 49 percent of the company and supplied the land, while Webb owned 51 percent and provided the building expertise. Boswell sold the land cheaply to the Development Company since he was to receive 49 percent of the profits made from the development of Sun City.

Webb's marketing and development strategy was to build community facilities before selling homes. He felt that "mature buyers" would demand a product instead of promises. Thus, before a single home was sold, the following was completed: a motel with restaurant, a golf course, a recreation center with a swimming pool, a lawn bowling green, shuffleboard courts, an auditorium, hobby studios, meeting and card rooms, a shopping center, apartments, model homes, and a sales office. With these facilities, even the first residents were able to engage in activities from the beginning.

Before Sun City opened on New Year's Day, 1960, Webb initiated a national advertising campaign. The campaign offered a two-bedroom, $10,000, top-of-the-line home for whoever best named the town site. The name "Sun City" was selected and a couple from Oregon became the first residents of the new community.

The advertising campaign proved to be an immediate success. During the first three days of sales in January 1960, 272 homes were sold. At the end of one year, 1,301 homes had been sold and Sun City had a population of 2,500. Ten years later (1970), the population was about 15,000 and by 1980 the population was almost 50,000. Because the community was to house no more than 48,000, a sister city (Sun City West) was initiated in 1978 to meet the demand for retirement living. Sun City West, located two miles west of Sun City, is discussed in the "Future Plans" section of this case study.

Not only has the number of people and homes grown in Sun City, but the number of services and facilities has grown as well. By 1981, the following services and facilities existed in Sun City: 6 major shopping centers with over 350 businesses; 51 financial institutions; 7 recreational complexes; a hospital; 10 medical and health complexes; 29 churches and synagogues; and over 300 clubs and organizations. Sun City has truly grown into a self-contained city.

There were two significant events in the development of Sun City. The first of these occurred in 1968. Prior to that year, development had been geared to middle-income people and was located in the southern portion of the site. A major street, Grand Avenue, was the northern-most boundary of development. When Webb decided to expand across Grand Avenue, a change was also made in the type of housing provided. In response to the demand for larger and more luxurious housing, the new houses were generally larger and more expensive than those in the southern portion of the community. These new houses generally attracted more affluent people to Sun City. The differences between the areas north and south of Grand Avenue will be discussed in several sections throughout this case study.

The second significant event in the history of Sun City's development took place in 1978-79. By that time, virtually all of Sun City had been developed and it had reached its projected population of about 48,000. Consequently, the Del E. Webb Development Company began phasing out of Sun City and concentrating on the development of Sun City West. Since that time, DEVCO has sold all shopping centers, restaurants, and office buildings in Sun City. However, the Webb Corporation is still interested and involved in Sun City since it is also in the business of reselling homes. About 2,400 homes are sold each year in Sun City, representing a 7 percent turnover rate.

Philosophy

The philosophy underlying the development of Sun City was to provide both a leisure and active community in a pleasant climate for people to enjoy their retirement years. The concept of a retirement community had first been tried in Youngtown, Arizona, in 1954. Sun City was to become the first community for the "active retired."

The Del E. Webb Development Company (DEVCO) used several approaches in implementing the Sun City philosophy. First, DEVCO built a community of homes and leisure and commercial facilities designed to satisfy the daily needs of a "50 years old and older" population and foster for them an active way of life. Second, DEVCO provided these facilities prior to building homes. Third, DEVCO developed Sun City in close cooperation with residents so as to determine in advance their preferences for services and facilities. Fourth, DEVCO established architectural and design controls that assured quality buildings for Sun City. Fifth, DEVCO was able to attract to Sun City the needed businesses and health care facilities, and professional people and services. It also assisted residents in developing other facilities such as churches.

Resident Characteristics

Number of residents. The population of Sun City in early 1981 was 47,600. About 60 percent of its residents live in the northern portion of the community (Phase II) and about 40 percent live in the southern portion (Phase I).

Throughout its history, Sun City has experienced phenomenal growth. During the first decade, Sun City's average population increase was about 1,300 per year. The population figures in Table 2.4 illustrate Sun City's growth.

This rapid growth has not been without its consequences. In a 1980 survey of Sun City residents, "control of growth" was the most frequently mentioned problem in the community (13 percent). The second most commonly mentioned problem was "traffic congestion" (9 percent).

Admission requirements. The only admission requirement at Sun City concerns the age of residents. It is required that at least one person in a household (the buyer or spouse) must be 50 or more years of age. In addition, people under 18 years of age are excluded as permanent residents, with few exceptions. One exception is that children may live in Sun City with their grandparents as wards or in the event of family tragedies.

Socioeconomic and demographic profile. In general, the residents

Table 2.4

Sun City Population

Year	Population
1960	1,890
1965	7,335
1970	16,367
1975	36,548
1980	47,524

of Sun City may be described as young elderly. In 1980, the average age of residents was about 69 years. About 75 percent were over 65 years of age; 22 percent were between 55 and 64 years old; the remaining 3 percent were between 45 and 54 years.

The average age of residents has not changed greatly since the mid-'60s. In 1975, the average age was about 68.5; in 1970, it was about 67; in 1965, it was about 68.5 years.

A striking age difference is seen between the residents of Phase I and those in Phase II. In 1980, the average age of men in Phase I was 72.8 and that of women was 70.6. By comparison, men in Phase II averaged 62.5 and women averaged 64.7. These differences are due to the fact that Phase I was developed in the 1960s while Phase II was a development of the 1970s. Thus, the residents of Phase I for the most part have lived in Sun City longer and, therefore, have aged with the retirement community.

Most residents are married and living with a spouse. It is estimated that about 75 percent of the households are composed of married couples. However, of the single member households, women outnumber men by eight-to-one. Overall, about 53 percent of the residents are women. This percentage has remained fairly stable throughout Sun City's history.

Although the residents are heterogeneous in terms of religion, they are racially homogeneous. About 99 percent of the population are white while the remainder are black. There are 35 religious congregations in Sun City representing an array of denominations. Twenty-five of these denominations have built houses of worship (3 Catholic, 1 Jewish, and 21 Protestant). In addition, several sites are reserved for the building of churches or synagogues in the future.

The socioeconomic profile of residents reveals a diverse population although Sun City is characterized as an upper-middle class community. The average income per family in Sun City in 1980 was about $22,700. This figure has been increasing ever since Sun City opened in 1960. To illustrate this increase, the average family incomes at five-year intervals are shown in Table 2.5. It should be noted that the largest increases in income occurred after the beginning of Phase II development in 1968-69. These increases are partially attributable to inflation, but they also reflect the influx of more affluent residents.

To further illustrate this change in average family income after the beginning of Phase II, the family incomes of Phase I and Phase II residents are compared. In 1975, the average family income of

Table 2.5

Average Family Income

Year	Income
1960	$6,850
1965	$8,320
1970	$9,635
1975	$16,588
1980	$22,710

Phase I residents was about $14,000 and that of Phase II residents was about $17,900. This represents a fairly significant difference, especially when it is considered along with the age difference between Phase I and Phase II residents. (On the average, Phase I residents are about 6 years older than Phase II residents.) Thus, the residents of Phase I are older and have less money than their counterparts in Phase II.

As mentioned earlier, there is a wide range of family incomes in Sun City. The residents appear to have fewer financial problems than the retired population in general. For example, 24 percent of the residents have a net worth of $250,000 to $300,000. However, one household in five has an annual income of less than $10,000 and 45 percent of these have more than one member. By comparison, only 23 percent of the households in the entire Phoenix Metropolitan Area have an annual income of less than $10,000.

These income figures indicate that some Sun City residents have financial difficulties. The financial planning of some residents has been negated by the rising costs of minimum necessities. In addition, health problems often precipitate or contribute to financial difficulties. This situation is complicated by the fact that home ownership may exclude residents from receiving public assistance. The Arizona State Department of Economic Security sets standards of eligibility for public assistance. (Arizona does not participate in the federal Medicare or Medicaid programs.) By these standards, it is not possible to receive public assistance if one owns a home above a certain value. Since most Sun City homes are valued above this level, few residents qualify for public assistance.

Sources of income among Sun City residents vary from pensions and annuities to social security payments, interest on savings, and stock dividends. Some persons who retired on fixed pensions many years ago are in need of assistance, but few apply.

The residents represent a well-educated, professional group of people. About one-fourth of the women and one-third of the men graduated from college. The median education of all residents is a little over 13 years. About two-thirds of the residents are from managerial or professional backgrounds. The following chapters of retired professionals exist in Sun City: Retired Teachers Association (one); National Association of Retired Federal Employees (two); military personnel (two); one each of physicians, lawyers, engineers, and college professors; and a union club was recently organized.

The political affiliations of Sun City residents tend to differ from that of residents in the surrounding community. More than 80 percent of the Sun City residents are Republicans, while within the State of Arizona, the voting population is about half Republican.

Although most (87 percent) residents are completely retired, others are still actively employed. Most of those who work do so part-time and on a voluntary basis. Only 13 percent of the households contain an employed person. Of the working women, one-third hold clerical jobs while 40 percent of the working men hold professional or managerial jobs.

The health of the average resident seems quite good. Residents are active in recreational as well as social and cultural activities. However, there is a portion of residents who need medical or nursing assistance. There are two nursing facilities within Sun City and two more just across the street from Sun City. In addition, there are many residents who receive home health care and some who move away due to the lack of sufficient nursing care. Although this less healthy group is in the minority, it is, nevertheless, a noteworthy segment of the population.

Residential history. Nearly two-thirds of the Sun City residents live in the community year-round. In 1980, 40 percent were seasonal residents with 28 percent living there 9 to 11 months per year, 10 percent living there 6 to 9 months, and 2 percent living there less than 6 months. In the last 5 years, there have been more seasonal residents moving into Sun City. For example, in 1975 only 35 percent of the residents were seasonal. This may be a reflection of the more affluent people being attracted to Sun City of late.

The average length of time people reside in Sun City varies between the Phase I and Phase II developments. In Phase I, 68 percent of the residents have lived there more than 5 years and only 11 percent have lived there less than 1 year. By contrast, 51 percent of the Phase II residents have lived there more than 5 years while 10 percent have lived there less than 1 year. Again, in these figures there is a reflection of the relative ages of Phase I and Phase II developments.

Residents of Sun City come from every state in the Union. Most come from other places in Arizona, although many may be transplanted northerners. The next biggest market state is California, followed by Illinois, Michigan, New York, Minnesota, Ohio, Colorado, Wisconsin, Missouri, and Pennsylvania. In 1980, most new residents moved from Illinois (17 percent), California (13 percent), and Michigan (10 percent). Thus, even though most Sun City residents move from the upper Midwest, Sun City truly has a national market.

In a recent survey, reasons mentioned most often for moving to Sun City were the climate, facilities, security, and community cleanliness. Similarly, the residents said they like their houses, the recreation facilities, and the well maintained appearance of Sun City. The least important reasons for moving to Sun City were the price of homes, closeness to friends and relatives, and being away from the city.

Although most people remain in Sun City until their demise, some move away because of the lack of sufficient nursing care. It was estimated that 25 people per month moved out of Sun City in 1980 because of insufficient health-related supportive services. It should be remembered that the Del E. Webb Development Company did not intend to provide health-related services or facilities in Sun City. However, the residents themselves have attempted to organize and attract needed services and facilities. This subject is discussed further in the "Medical" section of the case study.

Level of activity. Generally speaking, the residents of Sun City are very active and heavily involved in the activities of Sun City. Community residents participate in religious activities, perform volunteer services, study in organized classes, attend educational and cultural performances and sports events, participate in sports, as well as in arts and crafts, and generally help each other. The Recreation Centers of Sun City, Inc. charters 144 clubs and there are many more that do not fall under the Recreation Center "umbrella." It has been estimated that about three-fourths of the residents use these Centers. Those who do not generally have health problems. In addition, the Sun City chapter of the American Association of Retired People (AARP) is the largest of the 3,700 chapters belonging to the 12 million member organization.

Another indication of the residents' involvement in Sun City is the large number of organizations and facilities started by the residents themselves. Residents have started the following: the Sheriff's Posse; the Information Referral Service; Pride, which strives to keep Sun City clean; Boswell Hospital; the Sunshine Services; and a new 350-bed apartment complex with a health care facility. Residents are also currently trying to develop a home health care service. These and other organizations are further described in this case study (see "Facilities and Services").

Sun City residents are also actively involved in the affairs of Phoenix and the surrounding area. Many of the clubs and organizations of Sun City donate money made from crafts, etc. to local charities. Donations in the past have been considerable. Other clubs do tangible work to help residents of the surrounding area. For example, members of one organization work as teachers in El Mirage, an adjoining town with a population primarily of migrant farmworkers. Sun City residents also tutor high school dropouts while members of other organizations help a local Indian school. In addition, civic organizations such as the Lions, Kiwanis, etc. are very active in Sun City for the benefit of the surrounding community. Sun City residents are also heavy voters. On the average, over 70 percent of the registered voters in Sun City vote in elections.

Sun City does not employ a large staff that would have an opportunity to interact with residents. Residents are largely independent and manage many recreation and activity functions themselves.

Staff. The Del E. Webb Company employs 814 people in Sun City. The Webb employees include salespeople, management personnel, maintenance personnel, construction workers, etc. Over half of the DEVCO employees hold construction-related jobs. To operate the recreation centers, the managing resident organization (Recreation Centers of Sun City, Inc.) employs 280 full- and part-time staff. The Golf Course Division of this organization employs an additional 230 full- and part-time staff. Other examples are the Sun City Library which employs 2 librarians and has 230 volunteers and the Sun City Museum which has a staff of 4 plus 140 volunteers.

Staff members are not allowed to live in Sun City unless they comply with the age limitations. Some employees are residents, but most commute from neighboring communities.

Housing

Size and mix of housing stock. Sun City contains a total of about 25,500 dwelling units. Of these units, about 70 percent are single-family homes and the remainder are townhouses and condominiums. Almost all units are individually owned by the residents. This ratio of about three detached houses to one condominium has been the planned mix in the development of Sun City.

An examination of the Phase I and Phase II developments reveals a change in the mix of housing types. In Phase 1, 82 percent of the 9,800 dwelling units are single-family homes. In contrast, only 66 percent of the 14,300 dwelling units in Phase II are single-family homes. This indicates a change in the housing demand from the 1960s to the 1970s.

The pace of Sun City's development has occurred at various rates. Housing construction was at its peak in 1978 when 3,019 houses were completed. The lowest yearly production of houses occurred in 1981 when only 428 houses were completed (this figure includes Sun City West). This reduction in construction is due to decreased demand. Elderly people are having difficulty selling their homes elsewhere, particularly in northern states, so as to move to Sun City. A DEVCO executive anticipates that when interest rates drop, housing sales and construction will accelerate.

Because Sun City is a retirement community, it was planned to meet the needs of an aging population. Most all housing units are one-story and public buildings have ramps instead of stairs. The kitchens and bedrooms are also equipped with an abundant supply of storage space. However, houses have a front step at the door and interior doors are not wide enough for wheelchairs.

Housing units in Sun City vary greatly in size and appearance. The sizes of homes range from 900 to 1,900 square feet with the average being 1,676 square feet. Lot sizes average about 7,000 square feet. The one exception to this is in the Rancho Estates neighborhood where homes are located on one acre lots with corrals for horses. Bridle paths are accessible from each of the lots that lead to the dry bed of the Aqua Fria River.

In terms of housing appearance, there are many different floor plans and facades from which to choose. Thus, the neighborhoods in

Sun City have a variety of housing styles and do not seem monotonous.

Since Sun City is 21 years old and has experienced continuous development, housing units vary greatly in age. More than half of the single-family homes are less than 5 years old and 80 percent of the townhouses/condominiums are under 10 years old. A more detailed analysis reveals differences in the ages of housing in Phase I and Phase II. In Phase I, the median age of the single-family home is 12 years; only 40 percent of the residents are the original owners. The average age of condominiums is 13.5 years and 44 percent of condominium residents are the original owners. By contrast, the average age of the single-family home in Phase II is about 6 years; 84 percent are owned by the original resident. The townhouses/condominiums in Phase II are on the average 8.2 years old and 26 percent are owned by their original residents. These figures indicate that the development of townhouses/condominiums seemed to precede single-family homes in both Phases I and II.

Costs to individuals. The initial cost of moving into Sun City consists of the price of the home one buys. A large majority of homes are valued in the $50,000 to $100,000 range.

Throughout the history of Sun City, the prices of new homes have been increasing. Table 2.6 illustrates the average cost of homes built at 5-year intervals. These figures reveal that prices started climbing rapidly after 1970. Although inflation accounted for some of this increase, Phase II also began at about the same time. As reported earlier, Phase II consisted of larger and more expensive homes than Phase 1. For example, many Phase I homes were built of concrete blocks while Phase II homes were constructed with wood framing. In addition, lot sizes increased from 6,000 to 8,000 square feet. As shown by Table 2.6, new housing costs increased 2.5 to 3 times faster during the second decade than the first. Furthermore, prices doubled in a recent 5-year period (1975-80).

A comparison of housing values of Phase I and II further illustrates the cost increases and differences between the two phases as well. In 1980, the median value of homes in Phase I was $54,000 and that of Phase II was $65,000. A more detailed breakdown of the distribution of housing values is illustrated in the next table. Table 2.7 demonstrates that Phase I has many more homes in the $35,000 to $49,999 range than does Phase II.

The monthly costs of living in Sun City consist of mortgage payments and a fee assessed by the Recreation Centers of Sun City,

Table 2.6

Cost of Homes

Year	Average Cost of New Home
1960	$11,120
1965	$15,540
1970	$26,150
1975	$42,607
1980	$94,315

Table 2.7
SINGLE-FAMILY HOME VALUES

Market Value of House (1980)	Phase I	Phase II
Under $35,000	5%	0%
$35,000-$49,999	36	7
$50,000-$74,999	53	74
$75,000-$99,999	5	17
$100,000 and over	1	2
Total	100%	100%
Median Value of Houses	$54,000	$65,000
Median Value of Townhouses/Condominiums	$42,000	$59,000

Inc. Few residents now have a monthly mortgage payment since many have either paid off their homes or paid cash for them at the outset. For these households, the only cost is the $42 annual fee per person for recreation center membership. This fee is charged whether one uses the recreation facilities or not.

Demand. The demand for housing in Sun City is reflected by sales records. Throughout the history of Sun City, sales have been very rapid. The turnover rate has been about 7 percent per year for the last several years. This means that about 3,400 homes are sold a year in Sun City. About half of those selling homes do so to buy a new home in Sun City. Currently, there are less than .5 percent of the housing units vacant.

In order to keep pace with the continuing demand for homes in this retirement community, the Del E. Webb Development Company has begun developing Sun City West. This was necessary because most all of the land in Sun City has been developed. Sun City West is discussed in the Future Plans section of this case study.

Facilities and Services (F/S)

Because of the large number of facilities, programs, and services available within Sun City, the following discussion treats the physical facilities separately from the services and programs. Most facilities have been provided by the developer; the services and programs, however, are largely the result of the initiative of the Sun City residents.

F/S facilities provided by Sun City. Probably the most spectacular of the many facilities in Sun City are the seven recreation centers. One center boasts Arizona's largest indoor swimming pool, its first indoor, air-conditioned shuffleboard court, and its only synthetic surfaced lawn bowling green. Another center completely surrounding an outdoor swimming pool is located beside one of Sun City's two lakes with a boat dock.

Not all of the recreation centers are the same size nor do they include identical facilities. In planning new centers, several things were taken into account: population growth, frequency of use of existing facilities, and wishes of residents determined through surveys. Over the years, the centers have become larger and larger. The newest center is built on 27 acres and includes 10 separate buildings. In combination, the seven recreation centers offer: lawn bowling greens (8), shuffleboard courts (72), miniature golf courses (4), studios for almost every kind of hobby or craft, horseshoe courts, pool and billiard rooms, card and meeting rooms, swimming pools (7), auditoriums (5), tennis courts (17), table tennis, handball courts, racquetball courts, and bowling alleys (2 with 16 lanes each).

All of the recreation centers were built by the Del E. Webb Development Company. To fund the construction, a fee was included in the price of each home sold in the community. Thus, the residents actually paid for the recreation centers through the purchase of homes. In 1960. the fee was $125 per house. By 1968, it had increased to $200, and by 1980, the fee had jumped to $1,550.

As the Webb Company completed and equipped each recreation center, it was deeded over to the Recreation Centers of Sun City, Inc. This organization of residents owns and operates the recreation centers. The organization has no indebtedness because the Webb Company had fully paid for the recreation centers and all facilities within them prior to transferring title. The operation of the centers is funded by annual membership dues ($42 in 1981) required of each Sun City resident. Dues are assessed to each dwelling, even if it is unoccupied or the occupants do not use the facilities. Additional charges are made to users of the bowling lanes and golf courses. The Recreation Centers of Sun City, Inc. has an annual budget of about $2 million.

Also provided in Sun City are 11 golf courses. Ten are 18-hole courses and one is a 9-hole course. All of the courses were originally developed by the Webb Company and then deeded to either the Recreation Centers of Sun City, Inc. or to private clubs. Three of the 18-hole courses are owned by private clubs. The other eight courses are owned and managed by the Recreation Centers of Sun City, Inc. – Golf Course Division. These courses are self-supporting through user fees.

Sun City has two major community-wide facilities: the Sun Bowl and Sun City Stadium. The Sun Bowl is a 7,500-seat outdoor, grass terraced amphitheater with a shell-type stage. A variety of performances are held there such as music by professional individuals and/or groups as well as local talent. The Sun Bowl was built by the Webb Company and later deeded to the Recreation Centers of Sun City, Inc. At one time, Sun City Stadium was used by residents as well as the Milwaukee Brewers baseball club. The Brewers are now the sole users and are under contract to conduct spring training there until 1984. Sun City Stadium is owned and operated by the Webb Company.

Another excellent facility in Sun City is its library. The library was established in 1962 as a non-profit organization. By 1981, the main library had 40,000 books and the branch library contained an additional 8,000 books. It is heavily used by residents. In 1978, about 14,000 persons checked out 450,000 items. The library employs 2 librarians and benefits from 230 volunteers. Financing comes mainly from voluntary tax-exempt annual membership contributions, gifts, and donations. The library is not tax-supported and receives no government funding. Its budget in 1979 was about $87,000.

Sun City has numerous other facilities that help make it an independent community. Among these are 16 restaurants, including 9 golf course and bowling alley coffee shops and 3 dining rooms in private clubs. (The remaining 4 restaurants were privately developed.) The Webb Company also built a 97-room motel with an additional 18 apartments. In addition, a 230-unit vacation apartment complex was built to provide housing for vacationers. Sun City also has its own post office facility.

There is one notable exception to the long list of facilities provided in Sun City by the developer: no elementary or secondary schools exist within Sun City.

Services/programs provided by Sun City. The services and programs offered in Sun City are quite extensive. Many of them were initiated by residents. One such service is the Sheriff's Posse. Many Sun City residents felt they needed more police protection than that provided by the three sheriff's deputies assigned to the Sun City area. Thus, in 1973, a group of 30 residents organized the Sheriff's Posse as a legal arm of the Sheriff's Office. Members of the posse are unpaid volunteer peace officers, deputized and trained by the Sheriff's Office. These volunteers are generally composed of Sun City residents who had served with a local law enforcement agency, the FBI, or the military. The posse does not make arrests or attempt to pursue or detain suspects. Instead, they notify the Sheriff's Office about problems and potential problems. In 1981, there were about 300 members in the posse. These members pay dues to join and they buy their own uniforms. The posse is supported by public donations and does not receive financial support from the government. Currently, the posse operates eight patrol cars.

The Sun City Community Fund, Inc. was organized by Sun City residents in 1966. It is a non-profit organization that identifies sources of help and makes this information available to those who need it. One of the organizations' goals is to maintain the Sun City Information and Referral Service, which helps to bring people with various problems together with those who can help. The Community Fund also uses contributions from local residents to support agencies such as the Red Cross and the Sun City-Youngtown Dental

Clinic, to provide emergency loans, and to provide funds to hospitals and nursing homes for some of their patients.

Residents have even organized services to help those who may suffer from loneliness. For example, there is the "hello group" that welcomes new residents to Sun City. There is also a Friendly Visitor program for those who are homebound or lonely.

Another resident-initiated service is the Handi-Capables Club. Its purpose is to plan program and recreational activities of interest and benefit to Sun City residents who have long-lasting physical disabilities.

The Sunshine Services, Inc. was also organized by a resident of Sun City. This organization provides residents of Sun City and Sun City West with sick room equipment free of charge, for as long as it is needed. The equipment in stock is valued at over $400,000 and was purchased with the donations from residents. It is estimated that in 1979, this organization saved residents over $743,000 in rental fees.

To help those residents who cannot cook for themselves, Sun City has a Meals-on-Wheels organization. It is a non-profit agency operated entirely by volunteers. Meals are prepared at Boswell Hospital and delivered to those in need at a cost of only $3.50 per day. However, contributions make it possible to deliver meals to indigent residents as well. Over 100 people are served by this organization daily.

With all of these help-oriented services in Sun City, one would suspect that most all residents who need help receive it. However, conversations with representatives of these organizations reveal this is not the case. It seems that pride prevents many of those in need from asking for or accepting help.

Sun City also has numerous services and programs that are not only "help" oriented. Among these are 149 chartered clubs that use the recreation facilities. In addition, Sun City has its own symphony. The orchestra is composed of amateur and professional musicians who present five concerts each season. There are also other music performances of professional musicians at various times of the year.

Various modes of transportation are available to Sun City residents. First, the Del E. Webb Development Company provides a bus service. There are three routes within the community, each about 16 miles long, and each runs three times a day. On the average, about 40 passengers per day use the bus service. In addition, there is a shuttle bus that runs the two miles between Sun City and Sun City West. Another mode of transportation is the privately owned golf cart. It is estimated that there are 5,000 golf carts in Sun City. Some non-golfers even own golf carts. For many, the carts provide an enjoyable, economical means of travel in Sun City.

The transportation system in Sun City is not without its critics. The Sun City Community Council has stated that transportation services need to be altered. The Council argues that a transportation system in a retirement community where few people are employed is used intermittently. Thus, the system needs to be flexible and low cost. In light of this analysis, the Council has recommended the following: 1) organize volunteers to use their own cars for a transportation service, 2) use volunteers to drive vans or buses, and 3) organize a dial-a-ride service. These ideas have not yet been implemented.

Some Sun City residents also complain about other services provided by the developer. Some feel the developer only considered property management and not the social-psychological needs of residents. For example, it has been pointed out that Sun City does not offer nutrition advice, crisis counseling, or adult day care services. Some residents have suggested that a social worker should be available to residents just as there is a program person to deal with recreation. Although these ideas have yet to be implemented, groups of residents are beginning to work toward their establishment.

F/S provided by surrounding community. Because Sun City is an unincorporated community, all municipal services are provided by either Maricopa County or private companies. For example, Maricopa County provides Sun City with highway and road maintenance, library services, planning services, and nine county parks, all located outside the boundaries of Sun City. Law enforcement services are provided by the Maricopa County Sheriff's Department which allots Sun City three deputies and patrol cars.

The Sun City-Phoenix Art Museum, a satellite of the Phoenix Museum, is located within Sun City. Established in 1975, it contains no permanent collection but displays loan exhibitions. The museum employs a curator, a part-time secretary, and two security guards. It also benefits from the voluntary services of over 140 Sun City residents. The museum is subsidized by the Phoenix Museum but also subsists on local donations and membership fees of Sun City residents.

Various religious groups have built houses of worship in Sun

City. There are 29 Protestant, 3 Catholic, and 2 Jewish congregations in Sun City. Many have two services on the Sabbath because memberships are so large.

F/S provided by private enterprise. Several services normally provided by municipalities are available in Sun City through private organizations. For example, water service, sewer service, and refuse collection are all provided by private companies on a contract basis to residents. In addition, the Sun City Volunteer Fire District has been serviced by a private company since it was established in 1966. The word "volunteer" is misleading since all services are provided under contract by Metropolitan Fire Department, Inc. (the nation's largest privately owned fire department). Currently, there are three fire stations in Sun City. No station is more than 2.7 miles from any building and no second station is more than 4 miles away. To fund the fire district, the County pays 60 cents per $100 of assessed property values in the District, while not exceeding 40 percent of the District's budget. The County cannot increase the amount paid by more than 10 percent per year. The remaining amount is raised by a tax levied on property in the District. In 1978-79, this tax was 38 cents per $100 of assessed value. The total budget in 1978-79 was $839,970.

Probably the most obvious examples of private enterprise within Sun City are the six large shopping centers. Although the Webb Company originally built and owned the centers, they have recently been sold to private investors or realtors. Each shopping center has its own Merchants' Association, which plans special activities. Currently, there are about 350 commercial businesses and 16 restaurants in Sun City. Nearby shopping centers in Peoria and Youngtown are also used by Sun City residents.

Sun City has a large variety of financial institutions. There are 16 branch banks and 25 branch savings and loan associations in the community. As of December, 1978, these institutions had more than $983 million in deposits. There are also 6 brokerage houses in Sun City. Numerous low-rise office buildings housing lawyers, accountants, and other professionals abound in Sun City. The community also has two newspapers (a daily and a twice weekly) and an FM radio station. The radio station broadcasts regular programming plus news of local activities and public service announcements once an hour. Finally, transportation between Sun City and Phoenix is provided by the Greyhound Bus Company (four trips daily).

F/S provided by Sun City for the surrounding community. Since

Sun City is a self-contained new town with a wide range of facilities and services, it is difficult to identify the specific services provided for the surrounding community. In general, most of the recreation facilities built by the developer are intended for the private use of Sun City residents. However, Boswell Hospital and the numerous commercial facilities within Sun City are for the benefit of residents of surrounding areas as well as Sun City. It is important to note that Sun City is not an isolated community. It is made up of people who are actively involved in outside community service as well as those who are content to focus their activity and energy within Sun City— just like any town or community.

Table 2.8 summarizes the facilities and services available at Sun City.

Medical Care (MC)

MC provided by Sun City. The nursing/health care facilities within Sun City have not been provided by the developer. Any such facilities are the result of efforts by Sun City residents, philanthropic organizations, or independent health care providers such as doctors or dentists.

MC provided by government or philanthropic organizations. Probably the most notable medical care facility within Sun City is Boswell Hospital. It is a 355-bed, non-profit hospital that was opened in 1970. Boswell Hospital is a fully equipped, acute care medical center that offers in- and out-patient and community-based services. It is associated with 236 doctors and provides ambulance paramedic teams as well.

Boswell Hospital was a result of the combined efforts of Sun City residents, the developer (DEVCO), and $10 million contributed by the residents, businesses, the Webb Company, the J. G. Boswell Foundation, and the Kresge Foundation. Sun City residents initiated the drive to build the hospital and were very active in the work leading up to its construction. The Del E. Webb Development Company agreed to build the hospital at cost for the residents and also donated the land on which it was built.

One of the out-patient services provided by Boswell Hospital is the Coordinated Home Health Service. This service works in conjunction with the Homemaker Service to provide nursing care, therapy, and housekeeping to lessen the necessity for long hospital stays. In mid-1981, there were 50 to 60 Sun City residents utilizing the housekeeping service and about 60 active patient families utilizing the visiting nurse service.

Boswell Hospital offers several community-based services. The hospital's Social Services Department provides counseling and coordination of resources for persons throughout the greater Phoenix area. Boswell Hospital is also a resource for community education programs. These programs inform residents about health, illness, disability, and ways in which they can improve and protect their own health, including more efficient use of medical facilities.

In case residents require constant nursing care, there are two nursing facilities within Sun City. Sun Valley Lodge, opened in 1962, is a non-profit facility that provides retirement living with health care. Its housing types include independent living apartments, sheltered care, and skilled nursing care. Housekeeping and three meals a day are included in the cost. The other nursing facility in Sun City, Beverly Manor, is a for-profit facility and opened in 1977.

In addition to health facilities, there are also several health-related services in Sun City. One of these is the Sunshine Services, Inc. This service supplies a wide variety of sick room equipment and appliances for the disabled without charge to the resident. Another such service is Meals-on-Wheels, which delivers meals to home-bound residents. Sun City also has its own branch of the Red Cross. In addition to emergency aid services, the Red Cross arranges free transportation for older and handicapped people (door-to-door) for medical appointments, food stamps, social security office visits, etc.

Sun City even has two services to assist the blind. One service is performed by Sun City residents for the benefit of school-aged blind people. The other is for the benefit of blind Sun City residents.

The service for school-aged blind people is the Recording for the Blind, Inc., which is part of a national, non-profit organization. This organization tape-records high school and college textbooks for the blind and physically handicapped. The Sun City unit of this organization has become one of the most active units in the country.

The service for the benefit of blind Sun City residents consists of recording recreational reading. Sun City residents volunteer to produce tape recordings of news and recreational material for persons who cannot see or cannot hold a book or magazine.

In addition to Boswell Hospital, Sun City residents have the use of two nearby hospitals. One is the Valley View Community Hospital in Youngtown and the other is the Maricopa County General Hospi-

Table 2.8

PROVIDERS OF FACILITIES AND SERVICES
(NON-MEDICAL)

Location	Retirement Community (Developer/Sponsor/Residents)		Governmental/ Philanthropic	Entrepreneurial
	RC Residents	Non-residents		
Inside RC	Sun Bowl Sun City Stadium Recreation Centers lawn bowling greens (8) shuffleboard courts (72) miniature golf courses (4) craft studios horseshoe courts pool and billiard rooms card and meeting rooms swimming pools (7) auditoriums (5) tennis courts (17) table tennis handball courts racquetball courts bowling alleys (2 with 16 lanes each) library golf courses (10 are 18 holes and 1 is 9 holes) motel (97 rooms and 18 apts) post office vacation apts. (230) restaurants (9-hole golf course and bowling alley coffee shops and 3 dining rooms in private clubs) sheriff's posse Community Fund, Inc.	Sun Bowl Sun City Stadium library bus service motel post office vacation apts.	churches (35) police Sun City/ Phoenix Art Museum	fire protection water service 6 shopping centers (350 shops) professional offices 16 branch banks 25 branch savings and loan assns. 6 brokerage houses 2 local newspapers FM radio station 4 restaurants

Table 2.8
(Continued)

Location	Retirement Community (Developer/Sponsor/Residents)		Governmental/ Philanthropic	Entrepreneurial
	RC Residents	Non-residents		
	"Hello" group Red Cross Information and Referral Service Friendly Visitor Program 144 charter clubs Sun City Symphony Meals-on-Wheels Sunshine Services Handi-capables Club			
Outside RC			county library county planning building and safety services highway dept. services county parks	sewer service refuse collection 2 shopping ctrs. (Peoria and Youngtown) Greyhound Bus Co. (to Phoenix)

tal in Phoenix. Valley View Community Hospital is a 104-bed, full-
service, community hospital established in 1965. Since it predated
Boswell Hospital by 5 years, it was the first hospital in the area
available to Sun City and Youngtown residents. Nevertheless, most
Sun City residents currently utilize the services of Boswell Hospital.

Two nearby nursing facilities are available to Sun City residents.
Camelot Manor, opened in 1971, and Good Shepard Retirement
Center, opened in 1976, are located in Peoria, just across the street
from Sun City. One of these facilities is non-profit while the other is
a for-profit organization.

The Sun City-Youngtown People's Dental Center is a non-profit
health facility located in Youngtown. It is staffed by retired dentists
who work without compensation to provide dental care for the indi-
gent population of the area. This is the first facility of its kind in
Arizona.

In 1980, the Sun City Area Community Council conducted a
study of the nursing care facilities in Sun City, Sun City West, and
Youngtown. The study revealed that within such facilities, there
was a deficit of intermediate care beds. Table 2.9 details the study's
findings. Based on these figures, it was concluded that more beds
were needed in the middle range of care. Similarly, it was concluded that an additional 1,417 nursing beds were needed. Because
of these deficiencies in the number of nursing beds or other supportive services, it was estimated that about 25 people leave Sun City
every month.

Table 2.9

Available Nursing Beds

Independent Living   =   542 beds
Congregate Housing   =   73 beds
Personal Care   =   155 beds
Intermediate Care   =   165 beds
(long-term)
Skilled Nursing Care =   293 beds

Total   = 1,228 beds

The Community Council study also said that adult day care services were needed in Sun City. These services are required primarily for the frail elderly and would provide both health-related care and social stimulation. Staff of such a facility should include an RN, a psychological counselor, and physical, speech, and occupational therapists. The Council has estimated that there are 1,500 people currently living in Sun City who could benefit from the day care services.

To rectify these perceived deficiencies, the Community Council is currently working with the University of Arizona Long Term Care Gerontology Center to identify long-term needs in Sun City. This collaboration is to result in recommendations of community-based services for Sun City residents.

A group of Sun City residents is currently working to establish another life-care facility in Sun City. The People of Faith, Inc. has purchased 30 acres of land in the heart of Sun City from the Webb Company for the development of a 350-apartment life-care facility and infirmary. It is scheduled to open in 1985 and is being partially funded through donations from Sun City residents. By making donations, Sun City residents are guaranteed residency in the life-care facility. During the first 6 weeks of the fund raising drive in Sun City, $900,000 was raised. Bonds underwritten by Maricopa County will be used to finance the remainder of the construction cost.

Another group of Sun City residents, the Interfaith Services, Inc., is working to establish an in-home health care service patterned after the On Lok organization in San Francisco. The philosophy of On Lok is to keep people in their own homes for as long as possible by providing a range of in-home services including skilled nursing care. When the resident can no longer function within his/her own home, On Lok tries to see to it that an appropriate facility is available.

In conclusion, one of the few complaints about Sun City heard during the data-gathering visit concerned the shortage of nursing facilities and services. Some residents feel that the developer should have made more provisions for medical and nursing care earlier in the community's development. They argue that the developer was not just building houses and recreation centers but was actually developing a new town that is incomplete without the health-care facilities and services necessary to care for residents as they grow older. On the other hand, the developers argue that their business is building homes and facilities that revolve around active, resort-retirement living and that they are not in the business of providing health care related facilities. Furthermore, the developers have argued that by building nursing and medical facilities, the image of an active retirement community might suffer. This seems to be a crucial dilemma in the development of retirement communities characterized as new towns.

MC provided by private enterprise. Sun City has attracted many independent health care practitioners because of its large concentration of older and relatively affluent residents. There are five professional office buildings in Sun City that house doctors, dentists, and various medical laboratory facilities.

MC provided by Sun City for the surrounding community. The medical services and facilities that have been attracted to Sun City are generally not for the exclusive use of Sun City residents. The reader is referred to the preceding discussion of medical facilities for detailed descriptions of each facility and service. It is important to note, however, that Sun City is not an isolated community with respect to most of the medical services. For example, anyone is allowed to enter Boswell Hospital and anyone who complies with the age limits, etc. is accepted in the nursing homes.

Table 2.10 summarizes the medical facilities and services available at Sun City.

Ownership/Management/Governance

Type of ownership. Sun City has been developed by the Del E. Webb Development Company, a private for-profit company. Properties within the community are owned by individual homeowners and various private investment groups. Currently, about 95 percent of Sun City residents own their homes as compared to 72 percent of the Phoenix residents.

Type of management/governance. Since Sun City is an unincorporated community, it is governed by Maricopa County. The County has a five-member board of supervisors that serves as a governing and policy-making body.

Sun City does not have an official governing body. Instead, its residents are organized into several civic organizations that operate Sun City's facilities and services. However, these groups seldom work together to provide a comprehensive and consistent range of civic services since most have their own specialized interests.

There are five major community-wide civic organizations in Sun

Table 2.10

PROVIDERS OF MEDICAL CARE

Location	Retirement Community (Developer/Sponsor/Residents)		Other Providers (Govt./Philanthropies/Private)
	RC Residents	Non-residents	
Inside RC	Boswell Hospital education programs home health care counseling ambulance/paramedics Meals-on-Wheels Sunshine Service Red Cross Recording for the Blind	Boswell Hospital education programs home health care counseling ambulance/paramedics	5 professional office buildings with doctors, dentists, and lab facilities Sun Valley Lodge (nursing care) Beverly Manor (nursing care)
Outside RC			Valley View Community Hospital (Youngtown) Maricopa County General Hospital (Phoenix) Camelot Manor (nursing care) Good Shepherd (nursing care) Sun City-Youngtown People's Dentist Clinic

City: the Sun City Homeowners' Association, Inc.; the Sun City
Taxpayers' Association; the Retirement Center Association of Sun
City, Inc.; the Town Meeting Association; and the Sun City Condominium Chairmen's Association. The first four organizations
have similar purposes: to maintain the quality and character of Sun
City and to protect the various interests of residents. The Condominium Chairmen's Association assists the condominium boards
in management.

The Sun City Homeowners' Association is a non-profit organization founded in 1960, the first year of Sun City's operation. Its
overall purpose is to promote the protection of Sun City residents
with regard to their personal safety and well-being, their homes, and
the desirability of Sun City as a retirement community. The following are some examples of specific activities undertaken by the organization: 1) it helped obtain an adequate sewage disposal system
for the community; 2) it helps maintain Sun City streets through cooperation with the County Highway Department; 3) it promotes
resident compliance with deed restrictions; 4) it serves as an advo-
cate for residents in utility rate hearings; and 5) it helps resolve in-
equities in taxation, assessments, and utility rates.

The Sun City Taxpayers' Association, Inc. is a member of a state-
wide group working for the control of government spending and reduction of taxes. It has the largest membership in the state and takes
aggressive stands on issues such as taxes, real estate assessments,
fire protection, and water, sewer, and electrical rates. It also provides guidelines for those who wish to lodge protests to the Tax Ap-
peals Board.

The Sun City Condominium Chairmen's Association, Inc. is a
non-profit corporation whose purposes are to acquire and disseminate information and to advise its members on the operation of their
condominium groups. It also assists with legal and technical advice,
cooperative buying procedures, etc.

The Sun City Community Council was formed to identify social
service needs in the community and to disseminate information
about existing social services. Currently, it is working with the University of Arizona Long Term Care Gerontology Center on a survey
of local residents in order to determine their health care needs. The
results of the survey will lead to recommendations for new and improved community-based social services.

The Interfaith Services, Inc. is a new organization, formed in
May, 1981. Its purpose is to promote the physical, psychological,

spiritual, and social well-being of Sun City residents. Currently, it is working to establish an organization similar to On Lok Senior Health Services in San Francisco. On Lok provides a comprehensive continuum of care for older dependent adults who live in their own homes. Thus, it allows people to remain in their own homes for much longer periods of time.

The Recreation Centers of Sun City, Inc. is a non-profit corporation that maintains and operates the recreation facilities. It is managed by a nine-member resident Board of Directors who receive no pay for their services. This organization employs a staff of 243 full- and part-time employees to maintain and operate the facilities. The Golf Course Division employs an additional 230 full- and part-time employees to maintain and operate the golf courses.

Degree of resident involvement in governance. As stated earlier, the Sun City residents are a very active group. As evidenced by the number of civic organizations described above, many residents are involved in the various administrative activities of the groups. According to some residents, however, active members represent only a small percent of the total population. Nevertheless, the residents have been playing an increasingly active role in the operation of Sun City and its organizations over time. In fact, in many cases they have taken it upon themselves to initiate and organize needed services.

Financing

Initial costs. As stated in the ''History'' section of this case study, several community facilities were built in Sun City before homes were placed on the market. The cost of building these facilities in 1960 was $2.5 million.

Tax structure. Real estate taxes are paid to the County by homeowners and the property owners in Sun City. In 1978, the assessed valuation of real estate in the community was about $150 million and the total cash value of the real estate was about $850 million. In 1979, property taxes were $5.65 per $100 of assessed valuation. Thus, the annual property tax on a house with a market value of $40,000 is about $400 to $500. It should be noted that even though Sun City is not in a school district, residents still must pay school taxes. In Arizona, there is a state school tax for unorganized territories and a mandatory levy for the state's teacher retirement fund.

Some of the facilities in Sun City are or were owned by the Del E.

Webb Development Company. For example, until recently the shopping centers were owned by the developer. In such cases, the developer was responsible for property tax payments. It should be noted that the recreation centers were deeded over to the Recreation Centers Association of Sun City, Inc., which is composed of residents. Thus, the developer had no property tax responsibilities for the recreation centers after their completion. The Recreation Center Association is a non-profit organization and is consequently not taxed on excess income. However, the Association is required to pay property taxes on the land occupied by the recreation centers. This tax payment has been about $250,000 per year.

Sources of revenue. Revenue to develop Sun City largely came from three sources: 1) existing company resources, 2) loans, and 3) sales of homes in Sun City. Operating revenue came from various sources. DEVCO received revenue from the sale of houses and leasing space in commercial buildings such as shopping centers. The recreation centers were operated by annual dues paid to the Recreation Centers Association by each Sun City resident. Golf courses and bowling alleys receive funds by charging residents fees for usage.

Marketing and Plans for the Future

Advertising. The advertising for Sun City has taken various forms throughout the community's history. Before Sun City opened in 1960, Webb initiated a national advertising campaign. The campaign offered a two-bedroom, $10,000, top-of-the-line home for whoever best named the town site. After beginning sales of homes in Sun City, advertising was placed in national magazines that were geared to a retirement-aged readership.

Another form of advertising involved a vacation offer in Sun City. The Visitor Vacation Plan offered visitors a 1- or 2-week vacation in Sun City during which time people could see what it would be like to live there. Visitors were allowed the use of the recreation facilities, golf, bowling, and a few meals and lived in a group of vacation apartments built especially for this purpose. Also available to visitors were 19 model homes built on a mini-boulevard. Visitors could borrow a golf cart and browse through the model homes at their convenience. This vacation plan continues today.

The advertising for Sun City stopped in 1978, since development in the community was nearly complete. Sun City is so well known that word-of-mouth advertising is more than sufficient to attract prospective buyers.

The current advertising thrust of the Del E. Webb Development Company focuses on Sun City West, Sun City's sister community located two miles to the west. Sun City West opened in 1978 and is being advertised in much the same manner as was Sun City. Sun City West is utilizing a Vacation Special based on Sun City's Visitor Vacation Plan to attract new residents. In addition, a national magazine ad campaign is underway. Sun City West also benefits from the reputation and attraction of Sun City.

Future plans. In order to keep pace with the continuing demand for homes in Sun City, the Del E. Webb Development Company has begun developing Sun City West. Sun City West was opened in October 1978 and is planned to be another self-contained community. It is located on a 13,000 acre tract of land two miles west of Sun City. Plans call for Sun City West to be an unincorporated community and to offer services comparable to those in Sun City.

Sun City West is being developed in two phases. Phase I includes 5,700 acres and has a projected population of 32,500 people living in 17,000 dwelling units. About 85 percent of these units are to be single-family homes. Phase II of Sun City West is to include 7,300 acres.

There is one major change in the Master Plan of Sun City West as a result of the Sun City experience. Sun City West is designed around a main "hub" area where most major recreational, commercial, and financial facilities are to be located. In contrast, Sun City was designed as a series of neighborhoods, each with its own shopping and recreation center.

Plans call for Sun City West to be even larger than Sun City and, thus far, it has grown more rapidly than Sun City. In its first full year, it attained a population of 5,000, which is an average of about 7.5 additional residents per day. In early 1981, the population of Sun City West was about 7,000 people living in 3,600 households. The population figures shown in Table 2.11 illustrate the growth of Sun City West.

The people moving into Sun City West are generally younger and wealthier than those in Sun City. The median income of Sun City West residents is $21,900, which is much higher than that of Sun City. To illustrate the relative youth of Sun City West residents, the following breakdown of ages is compared in Table 2.12.

Table 2.11

Sun City West Population

Year	Population
1978	1,021
1979	5,231
1980	6,511

Table 2.12

Ages of Residents

Ages	Sun City	Sun City West
Over 65	75%	42%
55-64	22	52
45-54	3	5

Sun City West already has an extensive supply of community facilities. The most spectacular of these is a huge complex for recreational sports, physical conditioning, and creative arts. The complex cost about $6 million and is situated on a 47-acre site. It is the largest private facility of its kind in the Southwest. Sun City West residents pay an annual fee of $75 per person to support the center. It contains the following: a swimming pool, a jacuzzi pool, two indoor therapy pools, a physical fitness room, a 24-lane bowling pavilion, a 25-table billiard hall, ten indoor shuffleboard courts, a tennis gallery, eight platform tennis courts, 15 tennis courts, two handball courts, volleyball and badminton courts, four regulation lawn bowling greens, an 18-hole miniature golf course, a quarter-mile running track, a croquet court, and an electric game arcade. Plans call for two additional neighborhood satellite recreation centers in Sun City West as the population grows.

In addition to the recreation center, Sun City West has four 18-hole golf courses (two of which are private clubs). One of these courses hosts the LPGA $100,000 Sun City Classic. There are also two more 18-hole courses planned to be developed as the population increases.

Other facilities in Sun City West are the Sun Dome and a library. The Sun Dome is a 6,800-seat, enclosed auditorium for the performing arts. It is the largest facility of its kind in Arizona. The library has space for 40,000 volumes plus a reference and periodical section.

Medical services are provided in the Sun City West Medical Building. It is well staffed and is expanding services rapidly. The developer is also allocating land for a nursing home and an extended care facility.

Shopping needs are provided by Sun City West's own shopping center. It currently contains a supermarket, drugstore, clothing stores, restaurants, etc. Plans call for two more shopping centers in Phase I and a regional shopping center as well.

The homes in Sun City West are generally more expensive than those in Sun City. Homes in Sun City West range in cost from $65,000 to $130,000, with a median value of about $72,000. This compares to a median value of $54,000 in Phase I of Sun City and $65,000 in Phase II.

The cost of homes in Sun City West has been steadily increasing even though it has only a short history. The figures in Table 2.13 illustrate this increase. Sun City West also has two models of very expensive homes ($300,000). These homes are designed to attract the California market, who need to buy an expensive home to protect

Table 2.13

Cost of Sun City West Homes

Year	Average Cost
1978	$57,706
1979	$77,248
1980	$87,499

from heavy taxation their capital gains made from the sale of their California homes.

Even though Sun City and Sun City West are both designed to be independent communities, the residents of the two interact on a social basis. Many of the social clubs and organizations draw members from both communities. There is also informal social interaction between residents of the two communities. One exception to this interaction concerns the recreation centers. The recreation centers of Sun City and Sun City West are completely independent of each other. Residents of Sun City are not members of the Sun City West Recreation Centers' Association and vice versa. Despite the recreation center separation, however, residents of Sun City and Sun City West are increasingly considering the two communities as one.

The completion time of Phase I of Sun City West was initially estimated at seven to nine years. However, the high cost of money and a sluggish economy have extended this time to an estimated ten years. The construction costs of Phase I are expected to exceed one billion dollars. In addition, the development of Sun City West will mean hundreds of millions of dollars in new taxable wealth to Arizona and Maricopa County.

Overview—Impacts of Change

Effects of change in Sun City. Sun City has had an impact not only on the immediate region and Arizona but also on the country, and even on other countries. Millions of visitors have visited Sun City from all over the United States and many places throughout the world. Among these visitors have been representatives of governments, large corporations, and community developers. Many visitors have studied it and even tried to copy it. As a result, there are now cities named Sun City in Australia and Africa.

In the local area, Sun City has had an enormous economic effect. To begin with, over $1.25 billion in homes at original cost have been sold in Sun City. Furthermore, Sun City residents spend about $450,000 annually in the area. Residents not only spend money but also create jobs as well. Statistics indicate that one job is created in the area by every six Sun City residents (about 8,000 jobs). There are very few large companies in Arizona with as many employees.

The local financial institutions of the Phoenix region have benefited from the presence of Sun City. In 1981, the seven branch banks and savings and loans located in Sun City and Sun City West had deposits of $1.4 billion. This is up from the total deposits of $980 million in 1978. To illustrate the significance of these figures, the 1978 deposits represented 8 percent of Arizona's total savings dollars in Sun City, which contains 2 percent of the state's population. Furthermore, fewer than 10 percent of the Sun City residents obtained a loan in 1978.

Although there is a build-up of retirement communities in the Phoenix area, it is largely occurring in the eastern portion of the region around Mesa. Other than Sun City West, no new retirement communities have been built in the western part of the Phoenix area.

One of the few negative impacts of Sun City has concerned local school bond issue voting patterns. Sun City was originally part of the Peoria School District of Peoria, a town of 13,000 residents to the south. As the population of Sun City grew, more voters rejected requests for school bondage. Consequently, 12 out of 15 new building bond issues in the district were defeated by the more populous votes of Sun City and Youngtown residents. Thus, in 1975 Sun City was taken out of the Peoria School District as a result of petitions from both Peoria and Sun City. Although this action was favored by most Sun City residents, it represents an embarrassment in the history of Sun City to many residents who feel it was their civic duty to support the local schools.

Summary

Opened in 1960, Sun City was the first retirement "new town" developed in the U.S. Since then, it has grown to a size of nearly 50,000 residents and its "sister" community, Sun City West, was opened in 1978 to accommodate still further demand for housing.

There were two significant events in the development of Sun City. The first occurred in 1968 when the second phase of development began. The second phase differed from the first in that it was geared toward a more affluent population. The second significant event in Sun City's history occurred in 1978-79. By that time, virtually all of Sun City had been developed and it had reached its projected population of about 48,000. Since then DEVCO has been developing Sun City West.

In conclusion, it is safe to say that Sun City represents one of the richest sources of information in the world concerning the development and evolution of a retirement community characterized as a "new town." Its history allows us to examine what happens when residents age and have different needs than those which attracted them to the community in the first place. Furthermore, its success over the past 20 years provides information concerning successful developmental practices during uncertain economic times. Sun City does seem to be what it claims—"the standard of the world in resort retirement living."

Chapter 3

Retirement Villages

HAWTHORNE
LEESBURG¹, FLORIDA

General Description

Hawthorne is a privately developed "village" consisting of owner-occupied mobile homes on lots leased from the developer, the Colonial Penn Insurance Company. Opened in 1973, the community has no medical nor commercial facilities and has no age restrictions for residency. A site plan of Hawthorne is illustrated in Figure 3.1.

Location. Hawthorne is located five miles outside of Leesburg, Florida. Leesburg is in Lake County in central Florida, about one hour inland from both the Gulf of Mexico and the Atlantic Ocean. Access to major population centers is easy because of three major highways which pass through the County. By automobile, Orlando is 45 minutes away, Gainesville is 75 minutes to the north, Tampa-St. Petersburg about 90 minutes, and both Fort Lauderdale and Miami are about 5 hours away.

The topological features of the area are low rolling hills, several lakes, citrus fields, and pine forests. The site for the community was selected because of its rural, tranquil character and favorable climate. Hawthorne is located on the Palatlakaha River which feeds into the St. Johns River by way of the Chain of Lakes. Through this waterway, it is possible for Hawthorne residents to travel by boat to the Atlantic Ocean at the mouth of the St. Johns River in Jacksonville, Florida. Hawthorne also contains three stocked ponds. The average year-round temperature is about 70 degrees and the eco-

---

¹Much of the information reported in this case study was taken from a dissertation by William Henry Haas III, *The Social Ties between a Retirement Village and the Surrounding Community,* University of Florida, 1980.

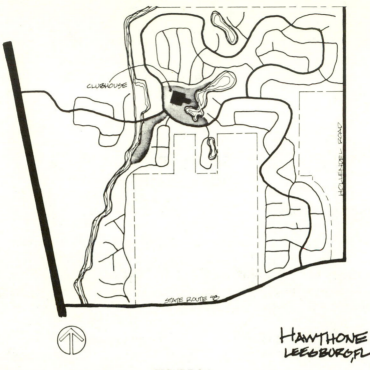

FIGURE 3.1

nomic foundation of Lake County is primarily agriculture (citrus). About half of the population of the County lives in unincorporated areas.

The area around Hawthorne has experienced above average growth in the past 10 years or so as compared to other counties in Florida. In 1980, the population of Leesburg was about 14,000 and that of Lake County was about 95,000. The average percent change in population between 1970 and 1978 for counties in Florida was 32 percent. Lake County grew 36 percent.

Lake County has also experienced a high rate of immigration. An analysis of the components of population change (natural increase and migration) reveal that between 1970 and 1978, Lake County had a -2.76 percent natural growth but a 100 percent increase due to immigration. Only seven other counties in Florida experienced large growth by immigration.

Lake County has a high proportion of residents 65 years of age or older. The County's elderly population grew by 78 percent between

1970 and 1978, while the State's increased by 58 percent. The proportion of elderly in Lake County was 21 percent in 1970 and 28 percent in 1980. This 1980 percentage is 18 percent higher than the national average and 10 percent higher than the State's average.

A regional map showing the location of Hawthorne is illustrated in Figure 3.2.

Size. Hawthorne is situated on an irregularly shaped, 300-acre tract of land. As stated above, there are three stocked ponds in Hawthorne and the Palatlakaha River runs through the property. In early 1981, about 2,000 people lived in Hawthorne; of the 1,200 developed lots, 1,150 were occupied.

History. Initial occupancy in Hawthorne occurred in October of 1973, but there were four phases of lot development. The mobile homes were initially sold from model homes and a plot map from which lots were selected. All facilities and recreation areas (recreation buildings, marina, etc.) were intended to be completed before the initial opening. However, construction was not completed until

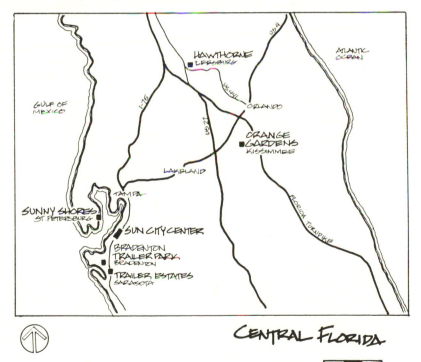

FIGURE 3.2

after the first 200 people had moved in (about 2 or 3 months.) Thus, these people were not charged rent for their lots until the common buildings were completed.

Hawthorne was the result of a request by the American Association of Retired People (AARP) that Colonial Penn Insurance Company build six retirement communities across the country. The relationship between AARP and Colonial Penn stemmed from the fact that Colonial Penn had underwritten the insurance for AARP for several years.

Hawthorne was subsequently developed by Colonial Penn as a pilot retirement community on which to pattern the remaining retirement communities to be developed. AARP was not financially involved in the development of Hawthorne. Even though Hawthorne proved to be a successful venture, the recession of 1975 and the high inflation rates that followed forced the abandonment of plans to develop future retirement communities. The president of Colonial Penn Communities, Inc. stated that development costs about doubled from 1970 to 1980. Thus, Hawthorne was the only retirement community developed by Colonial Penn out of the plan to build about six such communities.

Philosophy

The philosophy of Colonial Penn in the development of Hawthorne was straightforward. They strived to develop a community for secure and active retirement that would be affordable to middle-income retirees. Security was a priority because it was anticipated that most residents would retire from urban industrial areas in the North where crime was a concern. Thus, a manned security gate was placed at the entrance to Hawthorne. Opportunities for physical and social activity were felt to be important because the young retirees moving to Florida appeared to be oriented toward all forms of leisure. Thus, a wide variety of activities and recreation was provided. Finally, affordability was a priority so as to make it possible for a middle-income person to retire to a quality community in Florida. Thus, Hawthorne was developed as a mobile home community.

Resident Characteristics

Number of residents. Since it opened in 1973, Hawthorne has maintained a population close to capacity. Seventy to 80 people moved in immediately upon its opening and then 60 to 70 people moved in each month through 1975. In early 1981, the population of Hawthorne was about 2,000.

Admission requirements. Hawthorne has limited admission requirements. The only requirement is that no pets are allowed. There is no age limit placed on residency.

Socioeconomic and demographic profile. In general, the residents of Hawthorne can be described as young elderly. As of early 1981, the ages of people being attracted to Hawthorne have been in the 60s. The president of Colonial Penn, Inc. indicated that he would like to attract more people in their 40s and 50s. A survey conducted as part of a research project at the University of Florida revealed the mean age of residents to be about 70. The mean age for men was about 71 and that of women was about 70. Ages of residents ranged from 38 to 84 years.

The households of Hawthorne are mostly composed of married couples. About 84 percent of the population are married and about 14 percent are widowed females. Of the total population, about 55 percent are women. Generally, the widowed lost their spouses after they had moved to Hawthorne. Thus, most all residents move to Hawthorne as married couples.

In terms of race and ethnic or religious background, the residents are quite homogeneous. Most all of the residents are white, although voting records identified six "colored" voters in early 1981. Residents are generally Protestant with about 16 percent being Catholic.

The socioeconomic profile of residents reveals an upper-middle class group of people. They are well educated with the average resident having completed about 2 years of college. Prior occupations of residents include business, professionals, and teachers. A recent survey reported that about two-thirds of the residents rated their income as comfortable and one-third as very comfortable. Most all of the residents are retired and not working while living in Hawthorne. It is interesting to note that residents of the outside community view the Hawthorne residents as wealthier than they actually are.

The residents of Hawthorne view themselves as a healthy and active group of people. A recent survey found that a majority of residents felt themselves to be in good health and in excellent health for someone of their age. Twenty-three percent reported that they felt their health had actually improved since moving to Hawthorne.

Residential history. A large majority of the Hawthorne residents (about 83 percent) live their year-round. The average part-time or seasonal resident roughly spends the 6 winter months at Hawthorne and the 6 summer months in the North.

Since Hawthorne opened in 1973, residency has been stable. People usually stay at Hawthorne until their health no longer permits. From 1973 to 1979, the average length of residency was a little less than 4 years. Hawthorne's stability is further exemplified by the fact that there have never been more than 45 homes out of the 1,200 (less than 4 percent) for sale at any one time. This is a low percentage, especially for older people who would tend to have higher morbidity and mortality rates than the general population. The average percentage of homes for sale in other retirement communities like Hawthorne is about 10 percent.

A majority of the residents originate from the northern industrial states. Michigan, Ohio, and New York are the biggest market states. About 60 percent of the residents moved directly from the North. An additional 22 percent moved from other places in Florida. However, most of these were not natives of Florida, but had moved from the northern states.

Residents cite three major reasons why they moved to Hawthorne. The most often mentioned reason was security. As mentioned in the "Philosophy" section of this case study, security was one of the goals of the developer. The security system is expanded upon in the "Services" section of the case study. The second most commonly mentioned reason was the aesthetic beauty of Hawthorne. Hawthorne is a very well-maintained community partly because the developer (Colonial Penn) maintains the streets, mobile home lots, and the rest of the physical plant. The third reason cited for moving to Hawthorne was the recreational facilities and activities. These facilities are expanded upon in the "Services" section of the case study.

Residents generally move from Hawthorne because of deteriorating health and the need for nursing care; health care facilities do not exist at Hawthorne. Many former residents now live in nursing homes in Leesburg, while others have moved back North for nursing care, and to be near their children. In an effort not to move away, some residents have attempted to convince the Colonial Penn Communities, Inc. to provide health care in Hawthorne. These efforts have been to no avail, however, as the developer has repeatedly decided against such a change in development policy.

Levels of activity. The residents of Hawthorne are very active within the retirement community. Hawthorne provides numerous recreation facilities that help the residents remain active and out-of-doors. Many residents use the outdoor pool, pitch-n-putt golf course, shuffleboard courts, marina, and arts and crafts areas. Once a year the residents have a sale of the crafts made that year. There are over 100 clubs, classes, and athletic activities within Hawthorne. The recreational facilities are explained further in the "Facilities and Services" section of the case study. In light of this heavy involvement within Hawthorne, residents identify with Hawthorne much more than Leesburg.

Resident involvement outside Hawthorne is generally limited to matters that directly affect them. In general, there is a lack of interest in or limited understanding of the political affairs of Leesburg. However, some of the Hawthorne residents were instrumental in developing the proposal to obtain an additional nursing home in Lake County. Hawthorne residents also banded together to stop the establishment of a fire district which would include Hawthorne. Such a district would have increased taxes in the fire district to pay for the provision of fire protection. This was objectionable to Hawthorne residents since the retirement community provides its own fire truck. Later, the same fire district proposal excluding Hawthorne was adopted. This is clear evidence of political influence that the residents can and do mobilize when it is in their best interest.

Staff. Hawthorne does not employ a large staff that interacts with residents but rather a staff of 85 people. This is a resident-to-staff ratio of about 23-to-1. Most of the staff are maintenance people although there are also security guards, firefighters, office workers, and an activity director who has a staff of five. Thus, the residents are largely independent and generally only interact with staff related to the recreation facilities.

Most of the staff now live in Leesburg. Originally, the president of Colonial Penn Communities, Inc. had to bring staff with him from California because there were not many trained staff in Leesburg. Now, most of the staff are from Leesburg.

Housing

Size and mix of housing stock. The housing at Hawthorne is composed entirely of mobile homes. In early 1981, there were 1,200 lots developed, of which 96 percent (1,150) contained occupied mobile homes. The average lot size is 55 feet by 80 feet. All mobile homes are double-wide units and have two bedrooms and two baths. The size of the homes range from 1,100 square feet to 1,300 square feet.

Most were installed from 1973 through 1975 and are comparable in age.

Residents of Hawthorne own their own mobile homes, but they rent the lots from the management corporation. The management corporation also sells the mobile homes to residents. Thus, the management corporation is able to control the type of industrialized housing placed in Hawthorne and also maintain the visual quality of the site.

The lot lease contracts are guaranteed renewable to the residents and rent increases are based on the cost-of-living index as recorded by the U.S. Department of Labor.

Since residents do not own their lots but do own their mobile homes, the tax structure is affected. Residents do not pay property tax since they own no property. However, residents do have to pay a personal tax to the County on additions to the mobile home. This poses no problem for residents though since Florida is one of the least taxed states in the country.

Costs to individuals. The initial cost of moving into Hawthorne consists of the price of the mobile home. In early 1981, the average home sold for about $35,000. Typically, over 95 percent of the residents pay the price of the home in full at the time of purchase. Hawthorne is the most expensive retirement community in the Leesburg area, but the president of the management corporation explains that it also offers more for the money. Since Hawthorne opened, the mobile homes have appreciated at a rate of 5 to 7 percent per year. This appreciation is due to inflation and the high demand for housing in Hawthorne.

The monthly cost of living at Hawthorne is the lot rental. Payment of the lot rental fee allows residents the use of all services and recreation facilities except the marina which has an extra fee. Lot rental differs as to location and time of occupancy. In early 1981, the following rents were in effect; inside lot $179 (70 percent of the lots are this type); corner lot $186; man-made lake lot $229; and on-river lot $259. The president of the management corporation calculated that the average total monthly charge for residents in early 1981 was about $267 (including taxes, utilities, insurance, and rent). The value of each lot was estimated to be about $12,000 in early 1981.

The leases available to residents have changed over time. In 1970, Hawthorne offered a 3-year lease with a guarantee of no increase in rent of more than 15 percent during the term of the lease.

This was changed in 1975 to a 1-year renewable lease with price increases based on the cost-of-living index. This revised version of the base agreement has remained in effect to the present (early 1981).

Demand. Hawthorne keeps no waiting list for two reasons. First, the homes are owned by the residents and it is up to them to sell their mobile homes. Second, there are still vacant lots in Hawthorne (as of early 1981). Sales patterns have revealed the lots close to water and close to the clubhouse to be in high demand.

Adjacent to the 1,200 lots already developed, Hawthorne has another 113 lots engineered and ready to develop. These lots are to be developed when the developer feels costs to do so are more reasonable.

Facilities and Services (F/S)

F/S provided by Hawthorne. The services and facilities provided by Hawthorne are generally security and recreation oriented. Hawthorne was not intended to be a self-sufficient community. Residents are independent and must therefore shop and cook or make other arrangements for meals. What is provided, however, is a large clubhouse and a wide assortment of recreational facilities and programs that are convenient and free of charge to the residents.

Colonial Penn intended to have all services and facilities completed at the initial opening of Hawthorne. However, not all construction was completed before the first 200 residents had moved in and a method of compensation was devised (see "History" section).

Colonial Penn strived to make Hawthorne a very secure retirement community. There is a security gate at the main entrance which is manned 24-hours a day. Residents may operate the security gate by utilizing the electronic card readers. There are two other entrances to Hawthorne that are monitored by closed-circuit television. In addition to the security at the entrances, there is a security fence which bounds Hawthorne except at the western boundary which consists of a small river. The fence is a chain-link with barbed wire on top. And finally, Hawthorne has 18 uniformed guards who patrol the grounds.

The developer has also installed a security system in all of the mobile homes in Hawthorne. Each home has two "panic buttons" which, when pushed, notify the security office of trouble. In this case, a security guard and Hawthorne's own fire truck respond. Help can arrive anywhere within Hawthorne in less than 3 minutes.

All of the security guards are also certified emergency medical technicians. Thus, they are able to provide assistance until an ambulance arrives. This "push button" security system cost $300,000 to install.[2] However, the president of Colonial Penn Communities, Inc. feels it is worth it for the resident's sense of security and the advertising benefits it provides Hawthorne.

Other services provided by Hawthorne include maintenance, utilities, and transportation. Hawthorne is responsible for all grounds-keeping such as mowing lawns, trimming hedges, painting the lids of the underground garbage cans, etc. Streets are also provided and maintained by Hawthorne. Utilities provided by Hawthorne include cable television, water, mail delivery, and garbage pick-up. Transportation services provided by Hawthorne consist of bus service to Leesburg three times a week and to a major shopping center in Orlando once a week.

The recreational facilities and activities are extensive. Hawthorne has a large attractive clubhouse which houses a large auditorium, several small meeting rooms, and arts and crafts rooms. Outdoor activities include a pitch-n-putt golf course, a dozen lighted shuffle-board courts, a large outdoor swimming pool, a sauna and jacuzzi, and a 130-boat marina. All of these facilities are used extensively by the residents.

The only service or recreational activity that is not paid for in the monthly fee is the marina. Charges for the marina are $38 per month for a covered boat dock and $18 per month for an open boat dock.

Although Hawthorne provides these facilities for its residents, outsiders may use them if they are guests of a resident. The president of Colonial Penn Communities, Inc. indicated that he attempts to keep Hawthorne open to the outside because the residents tend to turn inward otherwise. An example of ways by which outsiders are encouraged to visit Hawthorne is that they were invited to attend a performance by the U.S. Air Force band which played in the Hawthorne auditorium.

F/S provided by surrounding community. Lake County provides Hawthorne with few services. Sewage treatment is provided by a regional sewer facility for which Colonial Penn paid a proportionate share of construction costs so as to facilitate the development of Hawthorne. Police protection is provided by the County Sheriff al-

---

[2]Not many other retirement communities have this system because of the cost.

though Hawthorne has its own security guards. Postal service and numerous churches are provided in Leesburg.

F/S provided by private enterprise. Private enterprise in the surrounding area provides Hawthorne residents with shopping, financial, and recreational services. Since Hawthorne has no commercial shopping facilities, residents go to Leesburg and Orlando for these services. Leesburg is close and convenient for grocery shopping and the like. However, Leesburg is a small town (14,000) with limited shopping. A recent survey revealed that the only aspects of living in Hawthorne that residents expressed dissatisfaction with were the shopping and lack of cultural events in Leesburg. Leesburg also provides residents of Hawthorne with banking services. In addition, there are six golf courses in the Leesburg area.

Table 3.1 summarizes the facilities and services provided at Hawthorne.

Medical Care (MC)

MC provided by Hawthorne. Hawthorne has no health care facilities although the security guards are trained as certified emergency medical technicians. In the past, residents have attempted to persuade Colonial Penn to add some sort of continuing medical care at Hawthorne. Colonial Penn has consistently rejected this idea because they do not feel they have the experience or expertise in the medical area to attempt developing a medical or nursing facility. Thus, residents must move out when they require nursing home care.

MC provided by surrounding community. Lake County has numerous hospitals and nursing homes. Of the four hospitals in the County, two are in Leesburg. Each has 135 beds. The other hospitals have 60 and 155 beds. Lake County also has five nursing homes. Two of these facilities have 116 beds each and the others have 82, 45, and 36 licensed beds. Leesburg has two of these nursing homes: 116 beds and 36 beds. Several former residents of Hawthorne have moved to the nursing homes in Leesburg. In this way they are close enough to friends for frequent visits. However, according to the president of the Colonial Penn Communities, Inc., Hawthorne has not affected the growth of nursing homes in the area to any great extent.

Lake County also has three home health care services. Two of these are located in Leesburg. These services provide personal care

Table 3.1

PROVIDERS OF FACILITIES AND SERVICES
(NON-MEDICAL)

| Location | Retirement Community (Developer/Sponsor/Residents) | | Governmental/ Philanthropic | Entrepreneurial |
	RC Residents	Non-residents		
Inside RC	security - med techs as well fire truck grounds keeping garbage pickup cable TV water mail delivery bus services to Leesburg golf marina shuffleboard pool sauna jacuzzi recreation all			
Outside RC			churches	shopping (groceries, etc.) banks post office 6 golf courses close by

(health aides) and skilled nursing care (registered nurses), as well as physical therapy, speech pathology, and medical social workers. Home health care services are available to persons who are homebound and are referred by a physician. These services make it possible for a person to remain in his or her own home much longer than would otherwise be possible. They also partially compensate for the lack of medical service provided by Hawthorne. Informal conversation with one of the home health care services indicated that there are several residents of Hawthorne who utilize their services.

Table 3.2 summarizes the health care services provided at Hawthorne.

Ownership/Management/Governance

Type of ownership. Hawthorne is a privately owned, for-profit organization. The owner is Colonial Penn Insurance Company who, along with the AARP, envisioned Hawthorne as a prototype for six retirement villages to be built in the Sunbelt. However, unstable economic conditions in the mid- and late-1970s limited development to Hawthorne alone.

Type of management/governance. Colonial Penn manages Hawthorne through a management corporation (Colonial Penn Communities, Inc.) which is a solely owned subsidiary of the Colonial Penn group. The president of this management corporation has the responsibility of carrying out the policy decisions of Colonial Penn and supervising the management staff who oversee the operation of Hawthorne. This staff consists of the following: a park manager who is responsible for the day-to-day operation of Hawthorne; a marketing director who supervises the marketing and public relations activities; and an activities director, who is responsible for the management of the activities of Hawthorne.

Degree of resident involvement in governance. Hawthorne residents have no formal role in govening their community. They do, however, manage and carry out the day-to-day operation of the approximately 100 clubs, classes, and athletic activities. Colonial Penn Communities, Inc. employs an activity director and assistants to help the residents manage the activities of the recreation hall. The activity director chairs a cabinet of residents who plan and organize events held in Hawthorne. There are also numerous specialized organizations made up of residents planning functions. The chairmen

Table 3.2

PROVIDERS OF MEDICAL CARE

Location	Retirement Community (Developer/Sponsor/Residents)		Other Providers (Govt./Philanthropies/Private)
	RC Residents	Non-residents	
Inside RC	security officers trained medical technicians		
Outside RC			4 hospitals 5 nursing homes 3 home health care services

of these organizations then report to the cabinet of residents for notification and planning of activities.

Financing

Initial costs. Colonial Penn invested $12 million in the development of Hawthorne.

Operating costs. To operate Hawthorne, it costs Colonial Penn Communities, Inc. $200 per lot per month or a total of $240,000 per month.

Tax structure. Property taxes at Hawthorne are paid by the developer, Colonial Penn, because the residents only rent their individual lots. In 1980, Colonial Penn paid Lake County $80,000 in real estate taxes and $14,000 in personal property tax (lawn mowers and other equipment). A 20 percent increase in these taxes is expected in 1981.

Sources of revenue. The $12 million invested in Hawthorne by Colonial Penn came from the funds of the Colonial Penn Insurance Company itself. Now revenue for operation of Hawthorne is generated by lot rental, and profits from sales and resales of homes. Thus, Hawthorne is now a self-supporting community.

Marketing and Plans for the Future

Advertising. In terms of marketing, Hawthorne benefits greatly from the connection between Colonial Penn and the American Association of Retired People (AARP) and the National Retired Teachers (NRT). A recent survey revealed that about 47 percent of the residents originally heard of Hawthorne through the AARP and about 19 percent heard of it through friends. The AARP and NRT advertise Hawthorne at exhibitions around the country and through mailings to their members. One result of this AARP connection is that Hawthorne has the largest chapter of AARP in the nation.

Although the AARP and word-of-mouth are the most productive forms of advertising, Hawthorne also utilizes television and newspaper ads. To concentrate advertising efforts, geographic areas are selected as targets. Generally, the northern industrial states such as Michigan, Ohio, and New York are targeted. However, recent civil unrest in the Miami area has prompted Hawthorne to advertise in that area with the result that one-third of all sales in a 3-month period in early 1981 came from south Florida. The Leesburg Chamber of Commerce Welcome Station refers people to Hawthorne as well.

To introduce prospective buyers to Hawthorne, tours are given year-round. It has been Hawthorne's experience that people visit two or three times before they decide to buy. They rarely buy on their first visit. In recent years, about 1,000 tours have been given per year with one to four people in each tour.

Future plans. In addition to the development of additional mobile home lots (see "Housing Demand"), Hawthorne also plans to develop land for commercial purposes. The residential development of Hawthorne is set back about a quarter mile from the major access highway. Colonial Penn plans to develop the land adjacent to the highway into small commercial concerns which would lease space from the developer. Thus, Hawthorne residents would have the convenience of shopping for their daily needs without leaving the retirement community. Construction is not scheduled to begin until economic conditions become more favorable, however.

Overview—Impacts of Change

Overall, Hawthorne has had a positive impact on the surrounding area. It has benefited financial institutions, while not overburdening the medical care facilities or drastically altering voting behavior in the area.

Economically, Hawthorne has attracted large amounts of money into the Leesburg area financial institutions and increased the tax base of Lake County as well. Hawthorne has been responsible for about $10 million of revenue to local commerce. Despite this large amount of money being funneled into local commerce, hardly any businesses have opened close to Hawthorne (Hawthorne is five miles outside of Leesburg). Only one convenience market grocery store has opened across the highway from the main entrance. Leesburg area savings institutions have received about $21 million in deposits from Hawthorne residents who also seldom request loans. In terms of property taxes, the property of Hawthorne produces about 20 times the revenue it did as a citrus grove.

The health care facilities have also benefited from Hawthorne's existence. The residents of Hawthorne have a need for health care, are financially able to afford it, and do use it. Despite this usage, the health care facilities have not been overloaded. Thus, Hawthorne provides a clientele without taxing the system.

Politically, the party affiliation of Hawthorne residents is generally dissimilar to that of Leesburg residents. However, the voting patterns of the Hawthorne and Leesburg residents are very similar. Thus, the high rate of voter registration in Hawthorne has not changed the voting patterns of the area.

There have only been two political issues in which Hawthorne residents played a decisive role. First, the Hawthorne residents blocked the creation of a fire district which would have included Hawthorne. If created, the district would have been funded by a special tax. Since Hawthorne has its own fire truck, the residents felt that they should be excluded from the district. Although the district was defeated, it later was formed with Hawthorne being excluded.

The second political issue decided by Hawthorne residents concerned a zoning change to allow the construction of a large glass container plant. The proposed location of the plant was between Hawthorne and Leesburg. Fearing that such a plant would set a precedent for future manufacturing close to Hawthorne, the residents and Colonial Penn halted the plant at the zoning board. As a result, some residents of Leesburg accused Hawthorne of eliminating jobs and slowing progress. Another interpretation of this event is that Hawthorne represents a potentially powerful political force that cannot be taken for granted or exploited.

Summary

Hawthorne was opened in 1973 as the result of a request by the American Association of Retired People (AARP) that Colonial Penn Insurance Company build six retirement communities across the country. The relationship between AARP and Colonial Penn stemmed from the fact that Colonial Penn had underwritten the insurance for AARP for several years. However, AARP was not financially involved in the development of Hawthorne.

Hawthorne was developed as a pilot retirement community on which to pattern the remaining communities to be developed. Even though Hawthorne proved to be a successful venture, the recession of 1975 and the high inflation rates that followed forced the abandonment of plans to develop future retirement communities.

Hawthorne has remained fairly stable throughout its history with little expansion occurring after the completion of the phased development. Another 113 lots adjacent to the existing 1,200 lots already developed are engineered and ready for development. In addition, Hawthorne plans to develop land for commercial purposes. Construction of these additional developments is not scheduled to begin until economic conditions become more favorable, however.

LEISURE VILLAGE WEST, MANCHESTER TOWNSHIP, NEW JERSEY

General Description

Leisure Village West (LVW) is a "retirement village" consisting of clusters of two- to six-unit rowhouses of condominium ownership. Occupancy of these units is restricted to people 52 years of age or older. Leisure Village West provides extensive recreational facilities and programs but does not offer medical services to its residents. This is a walled community with 24-hour security.

Leisure Village West opened in 1972 and is currently under development by the Leisure Technology Corporation, a for-profit development company with nearly 20 years experience in the development of adult and retirement communities in the United States.

A site plan of Leisure Village West is illustrated in Figure 3.3.

Location. Leisure Village West is located in Manchester Township, Ocean County, New Jersey, about ten miles west of the Atlantic Ocean, 55 miles east of Philadelphia, and 65 miles south of New York City.

During the past two decades, Ocean County experienced remarkable growth. In the 1960s the population increased by more than 90 percent and during the 1970s, by nearly 70 percent. This was due primarily to the development of retirement communities and the subsequent in-migration of senior citizens.

According to Ocean County records, in 1976 about 7 percent of all developed land in the County was in use for retirement communities with nearly 20,000 dwelling units and a population of about 35,000. By 1979 both the number of dwelling units and the population in retirement communities had increased by nearly 20 percent.

Between 1970 and 1976, nearly half of the County's growth was attributable to the increased population of senior citizens. During this period, the County's population of persons 60 years old or older increased nearly 75 percent to about one-quarter of the total population. In 1976 about 30 percent of the County population was 55

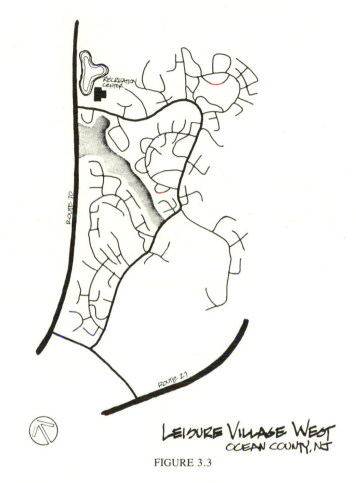

LEISURE VILLAGE WEST
OCEAN COUNTY, NJ

FIGURE 3.3

years old or older. Most of the growth occurred in the northern part of Ocean County, including Manchester Township. This area contains most of Ocean County's retirement community.

The construction of the Garden State Parkway in the 1960s opened Ocean County to developers. They were attracted by the inexpensive land, low tax structure, and the climate which is warmer in winter and cooler in summer than other parts of New Jersey and the New York Metropolitan Area.

By 1970, 40 percent of all senior citizen housing in Ocean County was in Manchester Township. In 1976, 20 percent of all developed land in Manchester was in retirement community use. Between 1970 and 1980 the township population increased nearly threefold and by

1981 it was one of the fastest growing communities in the State with a reported four out of five building permits given out for retirement community development.

A regional map illustrating the location of Leisure Village West is shown in Figure 3.4.

Size. In 1981, the population of LVW was estimated at 2,600 persons. These residents occupy nearly 1,600 dwelling units built on 240 acres. An additional 260 acres are for recreational uses while the remaining 300 acres are planned for residential use and have the capacity for an additional 1,628 homes.

History. Leisure Village West opened in 1972. It is the third active adult community built in Ocean County by Leisure Technology, a Delaware corporation. The corporation was formed nearly 20 years ago by a New Jersey builder who initially was inspired by Rossmoor Leisure World retirement community in Seal Beach,

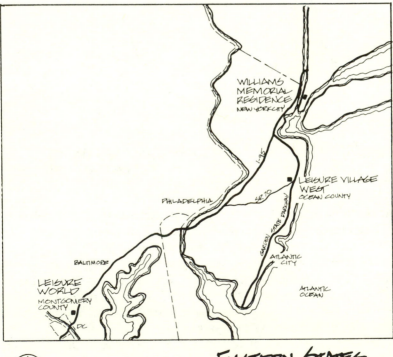

EASTERN STATES

FIGURE 3.4

California. He envisioned a scaled-down version of the Rossmoor community and saw the possibilities for marketing in the New Jersey, New York City, and Philadelphia regions with their relatively large Jewish and Italian populations. The rationale was that the groups tended to have strong family ties and many of the older persons would seek to live in an active adult community in close proximity to children and grandchildren. The first "active adult" communities built by Leisure Technology in the late 1960s were located in Ocean County. Their development and growth corresponded to the urban riots which prompted many New York City residents to look elsewhere for housing.

In 1974 the founder and then chief executive officer of Leisure Technology died. Changeover in leadership coupled with internal financial problems and periodic slowdowns in the housing industry and a faltering economy have impeded the continued rapid development of Leisure Village West.

Philosophy

The purpose or concept of Leisure Village West is comparable to all other retirement communities developed by the Leisure Technology Corporation. It is expressed in their advertising which describes a life of freedom from loneliness, fear, and boredom; freedom to choose from a multitude of leisure activities; and freedom from home maintenance.

Central to the Leisure Technology concept, especially but not exclusively for the East Coast market, is the proximity to one's prior place of residence and to friends and family.

Neither residents nor the developer consider their communities to be "retirement" communities; they are intended for "active adults" and are marketed for the middle class.

Resident Characteristics

Number of residents. In 1981, there were approximately 2,600 residents in LVW. Following the initial period of growth in 1974, about 800 people lived in the community. Within three years, the population increased to roughly 1,600. Its present population reflects steady if not spectacular growth.

Admission requirements. Leisure Village West is an age-restricted community. Eligibility is regulated by the Zoning Ordinance of Manchester Township. The community is zoned "Planned Retirement Community" (PRC) which restricts occupancy (not ownership) to persons 52 years or older. This person is called the "permissible occupant." A husband or wife of a permissible occupant or an adult residing with and providing physical or economic support to a permissible occupant may be of any age. Childen residing with a permissible occupant must be over 19 years of age.

Socioeconomic and demographic profile. The average age of residents is estimated to be in the early 60s. About 60 percent are married, 35 percent are single women, and 5 percent are single men.[3]

Most residents have a middle or upper-middle class professional background. Most are retired, while roughly 10 to 15 percent remain employed. Some workers have returned to work after retirement, others are working as consultants in the field of their former employment, a few are employed by the development company as clericals, hosts, and hostesses.

Leisure Village West is a community for healthy, physically active adults. No medical facilities are provided for the residents, who are expected to leave LVW when they can no longer live independently. Less than 5 percent of the residents are restricted in their activity by health problems.

Residential history. The majority of residents live in LVW throughout the year. About one-quarter spend the winter in Florida and other Sunbelt states. Some residents have second homes in these areas.

People move into LVW expecting to stay until they die. Roughly 5 percent of the residents move from the community each year.

Most residents had previously lived elsewhere in New Jersey. Since the opening of the community, about two-thirds of all new residents have come from within the State. In recent years, the proportion of residents coming from New Jersey and New York City has declined somewhat, as new residents have moved to LVW from other parts of the United States, most notably from Florida and the Southwest.

Residents are attracted to LVW by the security it offers and the ability to be close to family and friends. The recreation facilities, country-club living, and relatively maintenance-free existence are also attractions.

---

[3]Estimates of the mix of population are based on announcements of new residents published periodically in *Leisure Life News* published by Leisure Technology.

Residents leave LVW because of dissatisfaction with restrictions in the community, ill-health, loss of spouse, the attractions of a warmer climate or being near family, or for economic reasons. No one reason seems to predominate.

Level of activity. Residents of LVW for the most part are physically active. They play golf and shuffleboard, swim, garden, and partake in a wide variety of crafts, all within the community. The recreation director estimates that 60 percent of the residents frequently use the recreation facilities, especially for swimming and dancing, and that 5 to 10 percent never use them.

According to staff members, the newer residents are the most physically active.

Residents also participate in the operation of the recreation facilities. They sell tickets to various events such as dances, decorate and clean up for these events, assist as stage hands, monitor the shuffleboard courts and swimming pool, run the TV station, and assist in the greenhouse. All their work is performed on a volunteer basis. Resident involvement in the running of the recreation facilities is so extensive that the director's job has begun to diminish. The current director believes the position will be gone within 5 years.

Diversity of resident interest is reflected in the nearly 40 LVW clubs. These include service clubs, special interest clubs such as stamp and coin collecting, sports clubs (softball, volleyball), and activities clubs (bridge, gardening). All clubs are initiated and sustained by resident interest. Residents also serve on the nearly 20 committees to ensure the satisfactory operation of Leisure Village West (see "Ownership/Management/Governance" section).

Through their participation in LVW recreation facilities, residents have considerable contact with the recreation director. She sees her job as helping residents do what they want and defines herself as "very involved" with the residents.

Residents do not limit their activities to Leisure Village West. According to the recreation director, residents tend to use the LVW recreation facilities almost exclusively during the first 4 to 5 years and then they became involved in the surrounding community. For instance, many eventually join a country club.

Residents are active in the local churches and the local schools. Hospitals, an emergency first aid service, and the fire department also benefit from the money and hours LVW residents contribute. Residents have sponsored fund raisers for these organizations and the local high school band. They visit the high school on career days and referee sporting events at the grade schools.

Residents are also politically active. About 60 percent of the LVW residents turn out for local elections, reflecting their interest in tax and school issues.

Other than the recreation director, residents have little contact with other members of the management staff. There is little need for contact since all complaints and requests for maintenance, repair, or modifications to buildings or landscaping are handled through the appropriate committee.

Resident contact with the Leisure Technology staff is extensive from the time when the prospective resident first comes to LVW to look at a home until move-in day. The only need for contact after this is when there is some problem in the home that is under the developer's warranty.

Staff. In 1981, there was a sales staff of eight Leisure Technology employees at LVW. The regional offices of Leisure Technology were also located nearby. The Homeowner's Association (see "Ownership/Management/Governance") employs 40 persons, excluding security guards, to work in LVW. This is a staff-to-resident ratio of 1-to-65. The staff includes a manager, a recreation director, an accountant, and various office and maintenance personnel. Summer seasonal help is hired for grounds maintenance. In 1981 eight instructors were hired through the Recreation Department to teach various classes to residents. Instructors have always been hired from the outside rather than hiring Village residents but the recreation director anticipates this policy will change when the developer has completed construction of the community. All the staff members live in the immediate area.

Housing

Size and mix of housing stock. The entire Leisure Village West development is 800 acres. Permissible density, in accordance with the Manchester Township zoning regulations, is four units per acre. The developer is, therefore, permitted to build a total of 3,200 units on this property. This density changed after 1976. The original plan called for 5,000 units. This plan was changed because the developer decided to reduce the number of units to shorten the period of development, to build larger units in response to the market, and to accede to environmental constraints.

LVW is composed of 1,572 dwelling units in two to six plex, single-story buildings. Unit sizes have varied little since LVW opened, ranging from about 700 to 1,600 square feet. Most units have two bedrooms and two baths. Before 1976 one bedroom units were being built. Changes in unit styles have been made in response to market demand. In 1977 the developer introduced a new type of housing unit into LVW; all units opened onto open, green space rather than the streets. This was one of the innovations under the new management of Leisure Techonology.

Leisure Village West was planned by the developer for condominium ownership. This type of ownership is regulated by the condominium laws of the State of New Jersey. Each condominium is a cluster of buildings on given acreage and established under a Master Deed. For instance, during 1980, the developer was selling condominiums consisting of 92 units in 38 buildings. Condominiums varied in size from 18 to 31 units.

The purchaser of a unit in a condominium becomes sole owner of a particular unit. The owner of the unit also shares ownership of the rest of the property, the common elements of the condominium, with all other unit owners in that condominium. The common elements include the acreage of the condominium, the roofs and foundations of the buildings on that land, all improvements such as streets, sidewalks, and all natural features such as trees. Shared ownership also includes the garages and parking spaces of the condominium though each owner has exclusive use of an attached garage.

With the purchase, each owner becomes a member of the Leisure Village West Association which manages *all* condominiums in the development.

Condominium ownership carries with it certain obligations to the Association. For instance, individual owners must pay a monthly maintenance fee while permission from the Association must be obtained before any structural changes can be made to the condominium's buildings or landscaping.

The development of LVW has been slower than the developer planned both because of slowdowns in the economy and the changes in the company itself. In the first year, 1972-73, the developer predicted 200 sales of housing units since the community was new and relatively unknown. Based on the performance of the first two Leisure Village communities built elsewhere in New Jersey, the developer anticipated LVW sales to average 600 to 700 units a year, after 2 years. Both the Original Leisure Village and Leisure Village East were completed within 3 years. The Original Leisure Village sold 2,400 units or an average of 800 sales a year while Leisure Village East sold 1,400 units, an average of 500 units a years. Yet, in 1977, 4 years after it opened LVW had sold 900 units; by the end of 1980, 1,460 units had been sold. At that time, 240 acres or 30 percent of the land had been developed and contained a total of 1,572 housing units. The unsold units consisted of new housing and unsold housing from previous years. By May of 1981 all these units had been sold and construction had begun on new housing on the remaining 300 acres. The majority of the residents are satisfied with their houses and their relations with the developer. In a recent survey of new residents commissioned by the developer, 80 percent of them said they would recommend LVW to others. The other 20 percent responded negatively, saying they would not recommend LVW to their friends. They complained that their homes were not completed when they moved in and that when they were completed, they were not satisfactory. The new residents are among the most active members of the Homeowner's Association, a group formed in 1977 in response to dissatisfaction with the developer. An independent research firm hired by the developer found that nearly 30 percent of homes had not been completed as scheduled and nearly 40 percent were unacceptable to the residents. When the improvements were made about 35 percent of residents felt they were unsatisfactory.

Costs to residents. The purchase price of new units is set by the developer. Selling prices vary with the size and style of the units and on an average have increased by 120 percent between 1972-80. In 1972, units ranged from $21,000 to $38,700, an average of $25 per square foot; in 1980, they ranged from $56,990 to $73,990, an average of $70 per square foot. There is an extra $5,000 charge for a home fronting the golf course.

As stated above, each owner pays a monthly maintenance fee to the Association for the operation and maintenance of the property of each condominium and the property owned by the Association. Monthly fees are proportional to the size of the unit. The developer pays monthly charges on all unsold units.

Monthly fees based on single person occupancy in each condominium vary with the size and style of the unit. There is also an extra charge for each additional person. Monthly fees have increased as the community has grown and as the costs of operation and maintenance have increased. In 1976, monthly fees per unit ranged from

$34 to $68.75 and in 1980 they ranged from $52.50 to $106. The average fee in 1976 was $50 and in 1980 it was $80, a 60 percent increase. Fees for all units did not increase at the same rate, however. Monthly fees of units built before 1976 increased by only 50 percent; fees for units built after 1976 increased by more than 60 percent. There is an extra charge of $4 per person per month for units occupied by more than one person.

Owners also pay their own electricity, telephone, water, and sewage charges, and real estate taxes.

Demand. The demand for housing in LVW is reflected by sales which vary with fluctuations in the economy. In recent years, prospective purchasers of housing in retirement communities have had the same difficulties in obtaining mortgages as other home buyers. In LVW, this has not been a major problem since roughly three-quarters of the residents pay cash for their dwellings. For many, however, the greatest difficulty is selling their former home.

As mentioned above, the development of LVW has been slow relative to the development of the other two Leisure Village retirement communities which preceded LVW. Since the beginning of development, annual closings have been steadily decreasing. In 1973, there were 365 closings, in 1977 there were only 262 closings, and by 1979 there were only 120 closings.

The slow development of LVW has led to changes in the community's Master Plan. Each Master Plan change has indicated a reduction in the total number of units in the development. As of 1981, the developer planned a complete construction of the 3,200 units allowable under the current Master Plan and to build a second recreational facility.

Facilities and Services (F/S)

F/S provided by Leisure Village West. Consistent with the philosophy of Leisure Village West, there are extensive recreational facilities and areas available within the community. These include 24 acres with a 16,000 square foot activities building designed to serve residents from 1,750 units. It houses a kitchen, lounge, and an auditorium with a well-equipped stage. There are also dressing rooms with showers in close proximity to an outdoor swimming pool. There are studios for painting, sculpting, woodworking, sewing, ceramics, and lapidary, as well as rooms for cards and billiards.

Adjacent to the activities building is a well-stocked lake with row boats, two 9-hole, 3-par golf courses, eight shuffleboard courts, four horseshoe pits, croquet courts, two putting greens, a greenhouse, and a parking lot.

The recreation department offers educational programs, entertainment, and other social and sports events. For instance, there are classes in art, bridge, needlecraft, and languages. Instructors from outside LVW are hired to teach these. The recreation department also organizes trips to theatres in New York and brings in theatre programs, big productions, and variety shows. They draw from local talent for entertainment as well, for instance, the concert by the local Youth Philharmonic. Social events include dances with floorshows, barbeques, and pool parties. The recreation department also organizes tournaments for golf and shuffleboard and lessons in various sports.

The activities building, one golf course, and the swimming pool were built prior to construction of the first homes so prospective residents could see what was available. The second golf course was built in 1978 in response to resident demand. All the recreation facilities have been deeded over to the LVW Association by the developer.

There is a master TV antenna tower in LVW which is owned by the developer who rents the land from the LVW Association. The antenna serves LVW and other Leisure Technology properties in the area. Also available is a closed circuit CATV system which is used to provide entertainment and instructional programs originating from LVW to the residents. All these programs are produced by residents. One channel is reserved for continuous information on the schedule of events and activities in LVW and for emergency information. It is a primary source of communication within the community.

Leisure Technology publishes a newspaper for residents of LVW (and a neighboring community). The paper carries schedules of events, reports on club activities, announcements of new residents, articles on residents, and stories of general interest. It is also a source of advertising for local businesses.

Leisure Village West also provides its own transportation and security. The LVW Association owns, operates, and maintains a 44-passenger bus which was initially purchased by the developer and deeded to the Association. It is used to transport residents to major, local shopping and business areas outside the LVW. The LVW Association ordered a second bus for delivery in June, 1981.

Non-residents are excluded from this walled and gated community and must receive permission to enter. Guest passes are issued by the Board of Trustees of the LVW Association or a resident can call the gate to notify the guard of the name of the expected guest. To ensure the overall security of the community, the gates are guarded 24-hours by private security personnel and the grounds are patrolled from dusk to dawn by unarmed watchmen. There is little crime within LVW; at most there have been a few instances of petty theft reported.

This retirement community also provides its own grounds and building maintenance, street maintenance, and trash collection.

There are no commercial services within LVW. In 1981 the American Association of Retired Persons (AARP) Chapter of Leisure Village West was promoting the construction of a shopping center adjacent to LVW and the Board of Trustees was considering allowing a bank to open a branch office within LVW to be used by residents. It would also handle the payroll for the Association for a fee.

Water and sewer service to all condominiums are provided by the local township. Both the water and service plants were constructed by Leisure Technology Corporation and former subsidiaries of that company.

F/S provided by governmental/philanthropic organizations. Police and fire protection are available to Leisure Village West from Manchester Township. The police department is adjacent to the LVW property and they patrol the LVW community. The fire station is about one-half mile away from the entrance to the community. Both facilities were an integral part of the township prior to LVW.

A variety of recreational facilities are located near LVW including parks, golf courses, bays, lakes and rivers, public beaches, and picnic areas.

Since 1973, a bookmobile from the main public library in nearby Toms River comes to LVW once a week.

Since Leisure Village West is a private retirement community, the township in which it is located is not required to provide street maintenance or garbage collection.

F/S provided by private enterprise. Numerous facilities including shopping malls with national and local chains and specialty shops are located within seven miles of LVW. There are also numerous banks and savings and loan institutions in the immediate area.

Residents go to places of worship outside LVW. There are 15 churches of more than ten denominations within 10 miles of the community.

Until 1981, the only public transportation was a local taxi service. The Ocean County bus system began operation in the beginning of 1981 offering a 50 percent discount to senior citizens and the disabled. This service provides transportation from LVW to the shopping malls, government buildings, and hospitals. Various limousine services to nearby airports are also available.

When retirement communities began to be developed in the '60s, Manchester Township was predominantly rural. The increasing senior citizen population has stimulated the growth of nearly all businesses and services. This growth has been particularly great in the last 5 years. Most recreation facilities were already in existence by then because the northern townships of Ocean County have been resort areas since the turn of the century.

Facilities and services provided by LVW are summarized in Table 3.3.

Medical Care (MC)

MC provided by Leisure Village West. As in other Leisure Technology communities, no medical facilities are provided in LVW because to do so would be inconsistent with the image of an active adult retirement community. However, office space is available to physicians within the administration building. A private physician uses the space 2 half-days a week and by appointment, and a chiropodist uses the space 1 day a week.

Through their chapter of the AARP, LVW residents are organizing a medical clinic within LVW for use by residents. They received permission from the Board of Trustees, LVW's governing body, for their plan with the stipulation that the residents raise their own funds for the project. The plan is to have three to four registered nurses on the staff with the residents serving as volunteers. The clinic would be open 24-hours a day, 7 days a week. In 1981, shortly after Board approval was given, the AARP chapter had organized its first fund raiser.

Over the last few years a series of free medical lectures, given by doctors, was organized as one of the educational programs of the Recreation Department.

The primary contribution of LVW to the surrounding area is the

Table 3.3

PROVIDERS OF FACILITIES AND SERVICES
(NON-MEDICAL)

Location	Retirement Community (Developer/Sponsor/Residents)		Governmental/ Philanthropic	Entrepreneurial
	RC Residents	Non-residents		
Inside RC	activities building with: kitchen, lounge, auditorium, stage, crafts, hobby and game rooms, TV station swimming pool lake with boats shuffleboard courts(8) horseshoe pits(4) croquet courts greenhouse 9-hole golf course 2 putting greens newspaper security maintenance trash collection snow removal activities program trips		classes	
Outside RC		volunteers water sewage	police fire parks and recreation churches transportation recreation bookmobile	commercial financial

125

volunteer work and money the residents give to the local hospitals, the Hospital Auxiliary, and the paramedic First Aid Squad.

MC provided by governmental/philanthropic organizations. There are three hospitals located 7, 10, and 15 miles from Leisure Village West. One of these is a Class A hospital. During the '70s two hospitals expanded as a result of increasing demands, and in 1981 further expansion was planned by one hospital and a new hospital for Manchester Township was in the planning stages in response to the demand of the senior population. Various health and social agencies of Manchester Township were in existence prior to LVW, attracted by the numerous other retirement communities in that area.

MC provided by private enterprise. All medical services have increased during the 1970s in response to the demands of the growing elderly population in Manchester Township. Prevalent among these has been the construction of nursing homes in the area.

Medical facilities and services provided by LVW are summarized in Table 3.4.

Ownership/Management/Governance

Type of ownership. Leisure Village West is being built by Leisure Technology Corporation, a private, for-profit development company. The developer owns all undeveloped property as well as the unsold housing units in each condominium. Owners of units within each condominium also share ownership of the common elements of that condominium, e.g., the buildings, streets, sidewalks, and the plantings. The LVW Association owns the recreational areas, including the activities building and all developed community property which is not part of the condominiums. All community property, as well as recreational facilities and areas, were deeded to the LVW Association by the developer.

Type of management/governance. In 1972 Leisure Village West Association, Inc., a non-profit, non-stock corporation, was established as a vehicle for owning, managing, and maintaining all the condominiums, community property, and facilities in Leisure Village West. In the Master Deed of each condominium it is explicitly stated that the LVW Association shall administer, supervise, and manage that condominium.

The guidelines for management that the LVW Association is obliged to follow are established in the Master Deed, the Declar-

Table 3.4

PROVIDERS OF MEDICAL CARE

Location	Retirement Community (Developer/Sponsor/Residents)		Other Providers (Govt./Philanthropies/Private)
	RC Residents	Non-residents	
Inside RC	office space for doctors		lectures
Outside RC		volunteers	rescue squad nurses' registry nursing homes hospitals doctors health and social agencies

127

ation of Restrictive and Protective Covenants and Agreements, and the By-Laws of the Association.

The purpose of the Declaration is to "insure the continuance of a quality residential retirement community and to implement the provisions of the Condominium Act of the State of New Jersey." The By-Laws detail the procedures for operation of LVW by the Association.

The LVW Association is governed by a Board of Trustees consisting of no less than five nor more than nine members, each of whom will serve a 3-year term. Control of the Board is retained by the developer until October 26, 1987, which is 15 years after the date of recording the first Master Deed, or until all units have been sold, whichever comes first. Under New Jersey Condominium Law, 15 years is the maximum time a developer can retain control of a condominium. While in control the developer designates the majority of the members of the Board; other trustees must be members of the LVW Association and at least one of them must be a resident of New Jersey. The developer retains control of the Board in order to protect his interests and to teach the residents how to run the community.

From the first year until 1979 there have been three trustees appointed by the developer and two elected resident trustees. Then in the 1979 elections, in accordance with the By-Laws, an additional resident trustee was elected. This changed the composition of the Board to three elected resident trustees and four trustees appointed by the developer. According to the current resident trustees the decisions of the Board are nearly always unanimous. To help achieve this the current three resident members meet prior to each Board meeting to resolve any disagreements they have and thus present a united front at the Board meetings. Only one of the trustees appointed by the developer attends these meetings, with the proxies of the other three.

The duties of the Board include the operation, maintenance, replacement, upkeep, and protection of the buildings and common elements of each condominium, the recreational facilities, and all community property of the Association. It is also the Board's responsibility to estimate expenses in preparation of the budget, arrange for purchase of services and equipment when necessary, keep the books and maintain accounts, and enforce the rules. The Board may employ a manager to assist in these tasks. Because of the budgetary responsibilities resident Board members object to current practice of off-site bookkeeping. This is part of the impetus for allowing a branch office of a local bank to open in LVW.

The Board hires a manager to assist in the day-to-day operations of running LVW. The current manager was hired in 1972. Until 1980, his office was off-site. The manager's role has changed somewhat since 1979, with increased representation on the Board. Prior to that date the staff reported directly to the manager. Since then the staff has reported to the Board. Also, the trustees now approve all purchases whereas before the manager was free to make purchase decisions even for large equipment. According to one Board member, the resident trustees are really running Leisure Village West.

In 1977, two years before the formal beginning of the transition of control from the developer to the residents, some of the residents tried to gain more control. They formed the Homeowner's Association "to promote and enhance the general welfare of the community of LVW and its residents." From the issues they have raised it is clear that they are trying to have an input into the development and management of LVW and to guarantee their community becomes both what they want and what the developer promised. Their major complaint has been alleged poor construction. They have also objected to the developer's proposed changes of the Master Plan. After completion of about 1,200 units the LTC planned to switch from condominium to fee simple ownership in response to market changes. The Homeowner's Association resisted and 800 residents voted to form a separate community. The developer's control of the Board prevented this. They are currently involved in trying to correct alleged defects in street surfacing and to force the developer to build the second planned recreational facility because of overcrowding. These issues are also concerns of the residents on the Board.[4]

Degree of resident involvement in governance. Leisure Village West was designed to have extensive resident involvement. The Board, which has the ultimate power in running the community, will eventually be composed entirely of residents. All committees which oversee and advise in the various operations of LVW are composed entirely of residents. Neither the Board nor the committee positions

---

[4]In 1982 the Homeowner's Association was disappearing as various key members were elected to the Board.

are remunerative. The manager is hired only to perform the day-to-day operations of the community in accordance with the Board's policy.

In accordance with the By-Laws certain changes cannot be made without resident approval. All decisions involving capital expenditures require the affirmative vote of 80 percent of the members of the LVW Association and unanimous consent is required for the LVW Association to change from condominium ownership to any other type of ownership. Other decisions require a majority vote of the LVW Association members.

As stated above, residents are also involved in the running of LVW through the Homeowner's Association. Along with the issues already stated, the Homeowner's Association has tried to change the By-Laws, to loosen the landscaping requirements, and to establish each condominium as a separate, legal entity.

The Homeowner's Association claims a membership of nearly two-thirds of the owners. One of the resident trustees has stated that they achieved this membership figure through the sale of phone directories—anyone who purchased a directory became a member of the Homeowner's Association. This Board member estimates that about 20 percent of the owners are actually members. Nonetheless, the Homeowner's Association is an active group and a strong force in the community and turnout at their meetings is usually greater than at the LVW Association meetings.

Financing

Initial costs. Based on the front-end costs for other retirement communities developed by Leisure Technology, the initial costs for LVW are estimated to be around one million dollars. Besides the necessary land development these costs include the construction of the activities building, one golf course, and the pool. All this construction was completed prior to the building of the first homes. According to the developer, construction costs of homes have increased at the rate of inflation which averages about 1 percent per month.

Operating costs. The LVW Association maintains and operates all the property and facilities owned by the LVW Association and each condominium. It does not maintain or regulate the private property of the individual homeowner.

Maintenance includes painting and repair of buildings, mainte-nance of grounds and landscaping, and road repair. Operations in-clude the running of all the recreational facilities, payment of utili-ties and taxes, replacement of personal property of the Association, trash and snow removal, payment of insurance, and salaries. The budget is based on a yearly estimate of the costs of these activities. The yearly budget has increased both with the growth of LVW and with inflation.

In the fiscal year 1972-73 the total operating budget was $171,700 or about $860 per unit per year; by fiscal year 1979-80 the total operating budget had increased more than 600 percent to $1,212,245; however, the per unit costs had decreased by about 3 percent to $830. In the next fiscal year, 1980-81, the total operating budget had increased by 24 percent to $1,509,100 and the per unit costs had increased more than 20 percent to $1,000.

Tax structure. Property taxes are assessed by the Township of Manchester and the owner for each home pays the tax directly to the Township. Taxes on community property, recreation facilities, and the common elements of each condominium are included in the bud-get of the LVW Association and are paid from the monthly mainte-nance fees. Property which is owned by the LVW Association is taxed separately from all property owned by the developer. In 1979 the land owned by the developer was assessed at $1,672,200 and the property of the LVW Association was assessed at $569,900.

The taxes paid by the LVW Association have varied each year but there has not been a steady increase since the tax rate has also varied. In 1976 and 1978 rates dropped over previous years. Be-tween fiscal years 1972-73 and 1980-81 taxes increased nearly 25 percent, which reflects both a change in the tax rate and an increase in the value and amount of land owned by the LVW Association.

According to one of the resident Board members, the residents of LVW feel the taxes they pay are too high for the services they receive from the Township since LVW provides its own security, garbage collection, street lighting and repair, snow removal, and recreational facilities. The manager of LVW feels that none of the community facilities should be taxed. In an attempt to rectify this, Manchester Township is reevaluating its assessment of the LVW recreational facilities.

Sources of revenue. The monthly maintenance fees are the prima-ry revenues of the LVW Association. The fees are established by the Board of Trustees of the Association and are based on the budget required to operate and maintain the community. The projected number of units to be built and occupied for that year according to the development plan is used in estimating costs and fees. Each unit in a condominium, whether built or sold, is assessed a share of the total budget based on its share in the condominium. In essence, the larger the unit, the higher the fee.

During the first few years of operation, LVW was not large enough to bear the full costs of operation. To ensure a reasonable assessment of fees the developer assumed the payment of fees on unsold units. The developer has also subsidized an extra share of the total operational costs including security, street lighting, professional fees, landscaping, walkway lighting, and any other costs which increased with the development of the community. Also, the developer agreed to make up any deficit resulting from actual costs exceeding cost estimates.

The developer's subsidy has decreased each year of operation but the fees paid for unsold units have varied each year. In fiscal year 1972-73 the total contribution of the developer was $109,700 or more than 60 percent of the total budget. By fiscal year 1976-77, the developer's contribution had decreased nearly 60 percent to $45,800, less than 10 percent of the total budget, though in this year there was also an $8,000 deficit which the developer made up. During fiscal year 1979-80 the developer's contribution had dropped to about 1 percent ($16,900) but again there was a nearly $8,000 deficit.

Fee revenues from the unit owners have steadily increased each year. During the fiscal year 1972-73 these fees were $62,000; by fiscal year 1976-77 they had increased nearly 900 percent to $601,700; and by fiscal year 1979-80 they had increased another 100 percent to $1,207,295.

Other sources of revenue come from registration fees, guest badges and guest fees, e.g., for use of the swimming pool, and from miscellaneous income. Since 1977, this other income has been between $5,000 and $6,000 a year.

In December 1979, the first reserve of capital projects funds were established. These funds were set aside for roofing repairs for the condominiums and the activities building and for repaving roads. Then, in October 1980, a similar fund was established for replacement of maintenance and recreational equipment. These funds were instituted in response to a new New Jersey Condominium Law of

1979. They increased the monthly maintenance fees from $3 to $6 per unit.

Marketing and Plans for the Future

Advertising. Advertising for the Leisure Technology Corporation consists of newspapers, magazines, radio and television, billboards, and direct mail solicitations. New Jersey is their primary market but advertising also takes place in New York City and Pennsylvania. Leisure Technology's advertising approach has not changed since the community opened except to increase the volume during periods of slow sales.

According to Leisure Technology officials, the best advertising is word-of-mouth. They believe that most sales come from this source and that if the economic conditions were better, it would be the only form of advertising needed.

Future plans. There are approximately 550 undeveloped acres in LVW with 300 acres planned for housing and 250 designated for open space and recreational facilities. As of 1981, the developer intends to complete LVW's 3,200 units, the maximum units allowable under current development plans.

The developer is obliged to build a second recreation facility after the closing of the title to the 1,750th unit. If the developer decides not to build beyond 1,750 units there is no obligation to build the second facility. In 1981, 1,572 units had been completed and construction had begun on more units. If the present rate of unit completions and sales were to continue, the second recreational facility would not be built until 1982 or 1983. Construction could begin earlier at the developer's discretion, however.

There is tremendous pressure on the developer by the residents of LVW to begin construction of these facilities immediately. At one point construction was planned to begin in 1980, but slowdowns in the housing industry delayed this further. According to a resident trustee and members of the Homeowner's Association, most of the residents feel that the existing facilities are overcrowded. In the last 1 or 2 years there have been lotteries for dance tickets because the activities building was not big enough to hold all the residents who wanted to come to the dances; and in 1981, a guest fee for pool use was instituted to cut down on use. Yet residents know before they buy that the developer is under no obligation to construct the second facility until after closing of title to 1,750 units. This is explicitly stated in the public offering statement.

However, the Homeowner's Association considered the over-crowding to be so bad that in 1980 they brought suit against the developer, the LVW Association, and one of the developer's representatives on the Board over construction of the recreational facilities. In this suit they tried to halt further construction of units until the second recreational facility was completed. The case was thrown out of court.

The developer conducted a survey of residents to determine what they wanted in the new facilities. Tennis courts were in high demand and they are included in the current plan for the facilities. This second recreational area, if built, will cover nearly 28 acres. It will include an activities building, bigger than the current one, with an auditorium, exercise room, woodworking center, men's club, pottery and art studios, sewing room, first aid room, library, travel club room, and photographic darkroom.

Adjacent facilities planned include a swimming pool with whirlpool and patio, four shuffleboard courts, two tennis courts, two paddle tennis courts, a greenhouse and garden shed, an outdoor stage, and parking.

The developer estimates that construction would take one year and that the cost would be $2 million. The developer has said that the facilities would be conveyed to the LVW Association but the residents are concerned that the LVW Association will be expected to make a lump sum payment for them. There is also concern, expressed by a resident trustee, about the increase in the monthly maintenance fees that the additional recreational facilities will bring. It is estimated that fees will increase about $20 a month or a 25 percent increase and that from 5 to 10 percent of the current residents would not be able to afford this.

Some resident Board members anticipate being able to reduce operating costs when they have majority control of the Board and, therefore, the budget. They expect to achieve this through increased use of residents in the operation of the community. For instance, the Board plans to hire residents to teach classes in the Recreation Department.

On the other hand, the manager anticipates his position will become more important over time because residents will not want to spend their time running the community. He thinks the current level of resident involvement in the management of LVW is due to the developer's continuing control poised against the residents' increasing control of LVW operations.

Overview—Impacts of Change

Effects of change in Leisure Village West. Growth has been the major change in LVW since it opened in 1972. As the number of residents increase, residents report greater difficulty in getting to know everyone and a reduced feeling that they are a part of a community. The increasing population has also resulted in an overcrowding of the recreational facilities. As mentioned earlier ("Plans for the Future"), overcrowding has also led to an increasing demand for the second recreational facilities planned by the developer.

Effects of change in surrounding community. The development of Leisure Village West as one of many retirement communities in Manchester Township has been a tremendous stimulus to the local economy. Especially in the last 5 years there has been extensive commercial growth as well as the development of banks and savings and loans. The development has meant a continuing increase in property values. The construction of nursing homes, new hospitals and the expansion of existing hospitals has been a direct response to the increasing elderly population living in these retirement communities. The demand for these services will continue to increase with the development of retirement communities and the Township Administrator recognizes the responsibility of the Township to meet them.

This development has placed new demands on the sewage system. During the 70s two landfills for solid waste and a new sewage system were built. Numerous landfills have been capped and the County reports there has been some illegal dumping.

In the past there has been tension between residents of retirement communities in Manchester Township and other citizens of the Township over school bond issues. Retirement community residents, according to a Board member appointed by the developer, will support school bonds when they believe they are needed; thus local officials make a point of talking to retirement community residents and educating them on the issues. There has also been a shift in the locus of political power from the townships to the County over the waste disposal problems. Traditionally, the townships have been the primary political units deciding on zoning, approving development plans, assessing taxes, and so on. They see the need for the

County to establish the policy and find solutions for all the townships.

Both shifts in market demands and turns in the economy have impacted upon the overall design of LVW. For instance, according to a Leisure Technology sales representative, the company dominated the northern Ocean County retirement community development during the '60s and '70s. Then other developers started to come in and introduced single-family homes and fee simple ownership instead of condominium ownership. The response was so strong that Leisure Technology decided to change their product as well. It was in response to this that in 1977 they tried to bring fee simple ownership into LVW (see "Ownership/Management/Governance"). Members of the Homeowner's Association claim Leisure Technology tried to convert to fee simple because the company was in default and this change would release the company from the requirement of getting approval for changes on the Master Plan. The company did decide that all future East Coast developments would be fee simple single-family detached.

The prolonged development of LVW, due largely to the periodic slowdowns of the economy, had contributed to the tensions between the developer and the residents. According to the president of the Board, who was appointed by the developer, the delays have increased the complaints against the developer and the residents' expectations of the developer, beyond what is covered in the warranties. It is possible that this has contributed to the developer's pushing to close sales even before construction is completed. Findings by a research firm hired by Leisure Technology support this claim.

Leisure Village West residents identify primarily with their community, but, as seen, after about 5 years they become more integrated with the surrounding area. As the surrounding area has developed it has provided residents with greater opportunities to become involved outside LVW both as users of facilities and services and also in the development of those facilities and services. This has been especially true in the help that LVW residents have given to the development of the First Aid Squad and local hospitals.

Summary

Leisure Village West is a "retirement village" built by Leisure Technology Corporation (LTC). Its development has been protracted from slow sales due to periodic depressions in the national housing industry and from the death of the chief executive officer of LTC. In response, the developer reduced the number of planned units to shorten the development period.

The evolution of LVW is characterized by a change in the control of the community. Initially, the developer was in control of the governing Board. The transition to full resident control of the Board began in 1977. At first this was a time of disruption. Residents pushed to increase their control. Complaints against the developer increased. These conflicts spawned the Homeowner's Association. As resident control has continued to increase the turmoil has dissipated.

Chapter 4

Retirement Subdivisions

ORANGE GARDENS, KISSIMMEE, FLORIDA

General Description

Orange Gardens is a privately developed retirement "subdivision" in central Florida. It has no medical opportunities for its residents and limited recreational facilities. The housing is all conventionally built, single-family homes and there are no age restrictions regarding residency. Orange Gardens has the distinction of being the first subdivision in the country to be architecturally designed for retirement living. Since it opened in 1955, it has remained a clearly identifiable, unviolated, surburban-type neighborhood. A site plan of Orange Gardens is illustrated in Figure 4.1.

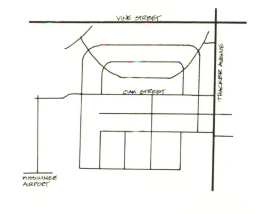

ORANGE GARDENS
KISSIMMEE, FL

FIGURE 4.1

Location. Orange Gardens is located on the edge of Kissimmee, Florida, which had a population of 14,500 in 1980. Kissimmee is about 10 miles away from Disney World and is included in the Orlando Standard Metropolitan Statistical Area (SMSA).

Kissimmee has been a retirement area since the 1940s. During that period, retirees came only in the winter months. There were so many seasonal retirees in the area that they formed the All-States Tourist Club. Membership was composed of retired people who lived in the Kissimmee area. The club is still in existence and many residents of Orange Gardens are now members. Currently, elderly people comprise about 30 percent of Kissimmee's population. This percentage has remained unchanged over the past 10 years.

Kissimmee is located in Osceola County. Until 1970, the County was largely a ranching area. In fact, Kissimmee was called the "Cow Capital" of Florida. However, since 1970, the population of the County has doubled to its more current (1981) size of about 50,000. This rapid growth is largely attributable to the Disney World development. Many young people have been drawn to the area by the lure of construction and tourism-related employment. To illustrate this point, Osceola County was the fastest growing county in the state in 1979. In addition, about 20,000 new jobs will be created in the next two or three years because of more planned theme-park development. Despite the influx of young people, however, Osceola County has a higher population of people over 65 years of age than any other county in Florida. About 20 to 25 percent of the County's population is seasonal.

The regional map in Figure 4.2 illustrates the location of Orange Gardens.

Size. Orange Gardens is situated on a 160-acre tract of land and consists of over 500 homes. In early 1981, the population was about 1,000, with 20 lots still vacant.

History. The development of Orange Gardens was begun in 1954 by Orange Gardens, Inc. Kissimmee had a population of 5,200 at that time and Orange Gardens represented the town's first new development in 30 years. The city was interested in the development of the retirement community from its inception and agreed to install sewers, water, and electricity. Streets were paved by the developer, but the city of Kissimmee agreed to annex Orange Gardens.

Kissimmee was chosen as the site for Orange Gardens because the developer wanted the retirement community to be near a city, but not in it. In this way, the retirement community could benefit

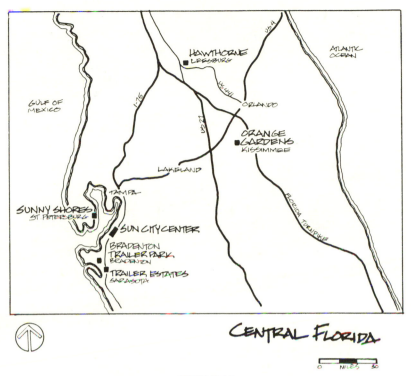

FIGURE 4.2

from the existing services, such as hospitals, shopping, and police protection. In 1954, Orlando had a population of about 100,000 and was close enough that Orange Gardens residents could utilize its service facilities. In addition, police and fire protection were supplied by Kissimmee. Thus, the residents of Orange Gardens were able to benefit from city services and facilities while living in a small town setting. The developer also felt that Kissimmee was a desirable location because it was not on the coast. The ocean was seen as a problem because it attracted too many people and metal products such as cars rusted at a very rapid rate. This location gave residents the opportunity to visit the beach, if they chose, but to live far enough away to avoid its liabilities.

By 1968, construction in the community was completed. The development corporation was dissolved in 1971 and the operation of Orange Gardens was turned over to a civic association composed of residents. The retirement community has now blended into the town as a whole with respect to construction and the age of homeowners. It is estimated that 15 to 20 percent of the homeowners are younger residents. It is important to note that after only 5 or 6 years of existence, Orange Gardens was thought of by local residents as a high quality subdivision, not as a retirement community. The developer views the assimilation of Orange Gardens into Kissimmee as desirable because it assures that Orange Gardens is an integral part of the community. In addition, it demonstrates that housing that is good for older people is good housing for everyone.

Philosophy

The developer of Orange Gardens felt that three criteria should be met in the design of a retirement community. First, homes should be planned and designed specifically to meet the needs of older adults. Second, the community should be located near recreation facilities, health facilities, shopping and transportation services, and a variety of cultural opportunities. Third, the community should provide a sense of purpose and status to the residents who are separated from their customary moorings of long-time jobs and familiar neighborhoods.

To meet the needs of older people, the homes were designed to be as safe and convenient as possible. The homes were also designed so as to be especially easy to maintain and have ample storage space. The special design features of the homes are described more fully in the "Housing" section of this case study.

It was also the plan of the developer to build different sized houses equal in quality. This was initially problematic because the lending institutions were reluctant to finance the low-cost homes. They believed that low-cost homes had higher than average maintenance costs. However, as a result of the Orange Gardens experience, local lending institutions now evaluate the quality of construction and not just price.

The developer also wanted to create a clearly indentifiable neighborhood that would become integrated into the existing town. He felt it was important for Orange Gardens to be sufficiently attached and part of an established urban area (Orlando) so that the living needs of an aging and retired population (social, cultural, and economic) could be adequately met.

The developer also decided not to impose age restrictions on residents of Orange Gardens. In fact, it was the intent that 15 to 20 percent of the population would be young families. These families were not segregated into a separate area of the retirement community, either. Thus, Orange Gardens was an age-integrated subdivision that was designed to be supportive of an aging population. It was also designed to be assimilated into the larger community of Kissimmee.

Resident Characteristics

Number of residents. In 1981, Orange Gardens had a population of about 1,000. This population size has remained fairly constant since construction of the retirement community was completed in 1968.

Admission requirements. There are no age restrictions or special requirements for admission to Orange Gardens.

Socioeconomic and demographic profile. The average age of residents living in Orange Gardens is rather deceiving since 15 to 20 percent of the households are composed of younger families. Thus, a percentage breakdown of the composition of households is provided instead. About 20 percent of the households are young families with children. In addition, another 10 percent of the households are young families without children. The remaining 70 percent of the households are composed of retirees who are 65 years of age and older. Among these retirees are a large number of people in their 80s and 90s. These resident proportions have remained fairly stable throughout the history of Orange Gardens.

A high proportion of the households are composed of married couples. There are more females than males, but not disproportionately more than the general population. The developer estimated that there are about 10 percent more females than males.

A socioeconomic profile of the residents reveals them to be white, middle-class, professional people. There are no black people living in Orange Gardens and only a few Asian people. Many residents are retired school teachers, but there is a wide assortment of vocational backgrounds among residents.

Many residents are living on low incomes. For example, teachers who retired in 1960-65 with retirement incomes have been adversely affected by spiraling inflation. One advantage of living at Orange Gardens for these people is that they own their homes. In addition, Florida's homestead tax exemption helps, too. Florida offers a $5,000 tax exemption off of the assessed value of one's home for the computation of property taxes. Retirees are given a $10,000 exemption off the home's assessed value. This exemption is about to be raised to $25,000, which will be very beneficial to homeowners, especially those on fixed incomes such as many retirees.

Several of the Orange Gardens residents still work part-time. About half work part-time and more than half engage in volunteer service. Some work in filling stations, as receptionists, and the like. These types of part-time jobs are fairly common for retirees in Florida. It should be noted that many people take part-time jobs not out of need, but to keep busy and earn a little extra money. The health of the retirees living in Orange Gardens is quite good. This is evidenced by the high percentage of retirees who still work part-time.

Residential history. Most residents live in Orange Gardens throughout the year. The developer estimated that there are only about 8 to 10 families (out of approximately 500 families) who are seasonal residents.

Orange Gardens attracts its residents from two distinct areas of the country. The strongest market is the midwestern states of Michigan, Ohio, Illinois, and Indiana. The next strongest market area includes Pennsylvania, New Jersey, and New York. Together, these seven states account for over half of the residents of the community.

Most people reside in Orange Gardens until their deaths. However, some do move away. Reasons given for such a move among the retirees revolve around health concerns. Some move because of the death of a spouse and others move when their health deteriorates. Some of the younger families move just because they want to try some place else to live.

Level of activity. The residents of Orange Gardens are an active group of people. Within the retirement community, residents have been heavily involved in the Civic Association, which is in charge of rules and regulations for Orange Gardens. Residents have also been actively involved in the Orange Gardens "Crime Watch" organization. The crime watch area was established by the residents in conjunction with the Kissimmee police to increase the security of the retirement community.

Orange Gardens residents are also actively involved in functions outside the retirement community. The residents have a record of being heavy voters. In fact, many of the city elections have been decided by the Orange Gardens vote. It seems that the residents of the retirement community are predominantly Republican while Kissimmee is predominantly Democratic. The Orange Garden residents also participate in the YMCA, suicide prevention, Council on Aging, Meals-on-Wheels, Red Cross, and the United Fund. In addition, a group of residents originated the County Art and Culture Center and actively participate in its operation.

Staff. Orange Gardens employs very few staff because the residents own their own homes and care for their own properties. However, when Orange Gardens, Inc. existed, there was a manager to help residents with various problems. Since Orange Gardens, Inc. dissolved in 1968, there has been no manager and the residents have run the retirement community through a Civic Association.

Housing

Size and mix of housing stock. Orange Gardens is composed of single-family, conventionally built homes. There are about 550 lots in the retirement community with only 20 of them vacant. There has been no active building since 1968. All houses were custom built for the purchasers. Thus, no homes were built until they were sold. Efforts were made to assure that no two houses looked alike by making various modifications on a group of general designs. The developer would also sell a purchaser a lot without a house. The purchaser could then build his own home at his convenience.

All homes built by Orange Gardens, Inc. were designed especially for older people. The homes were built barrier-free, inside and outside. To eliminate the step into a house, the developer ramped the ground up to each house. Thus, no step was needed and drainage codes were satisfied as well. In addition, the kitchen and bathrooms were specially equipped because these are the areas in the home where most accidents occur. In the kitchen, cabinets were mounted so as to minimize climbing and stooping. The kitchen counter was also mounted three inches higher than normal so a person could work without bending over (35 inches instead of 32). In the bathroom, all fixtures were bolted to wall studs for support. Handholds were mounted around the end and side of the tub and behind the toilet. Even the soap dishes and shower curtain rods were reinforced. With the reinforcement provided, all of these fixtures could support up to 1,000 pounds. Thus a person could grab any of the fixtures for support. In addition, the bathroom counter was mounted 5 or 6 inches higher than normal so a person could stand upright and use the wash basin. The toilet was also placed next to the bathtub in order to help the person get into the tub. With this positioning, a person could sit on the toilet, then swing his legs into the tub, and then shift his body into the tub. The tubs were also equipped with non-skid strips.

There were other special features in the houses as well. All electric outlets were placed 26 inches above the floor to minimize stooping. Baseboards were dark to provide contrast between the floor plane and the wall plane. Floors were made of terrazzo to simplify housekeeping chores. Terrazzo requires only a wet mop. And finally, all doors were made wide enough to admit a wheelchair.

In 1961, the wife of the developer conducted a survey of residents to determine what retirees really wanted and used in housing. The State of Florida called her study the most complete and authoritative study of retirement housing available at that time. The State also distributed the results to home builders and retirees. The study revealed that the features most approved of were the safety bars and non-skid strips in the bathtubs. Also liked were the wide doors, the easily cleaned floors, and the lack of steps anywhere in the house. According to the developer, these features made it possible for the wife to retire, too. Other features favorably mentioned were the accessible cupboards, the numerous closets, abundant storage, and the easily accessible electric outlets. In addition, it was reported that during the first 7 years of Orange Gardens' history, not one accident occurred in a bathroom. Yet, according to the National Safety Council, more accidents occur in the bathroom than in any other room in a house.

A seemingly potential danger of designing homes especially for older people is that they might not attract the younger residents, who were to represent 15 to 20 percent of Orange Gardens' population. However, this problem never developed. There were even two homes designed specifically for paraplegic residents. For example, no cabinets were placed under the sinks so as to allow for wheelchair access. When these homes were resold, the new owners never realized that they were specialized homes. Likewise, the resale of other homes in Orange Gardens has never been a problem because of the special design features for older people. Instead, Orange Gardens' reputation has evolved into one of a high quality subdivision—not a retirement community. Thus, the Orange Gardens experience indicates that housing that is good for older people is also good for younger people as well.

As stated earlier, the home sizes in Orange Gardens were intentionally varied. About two-thirds of the homes have two bedrooms and the remainder have three bedrooms. The houses also range in size from 750 square feet to 1,700 square feet. The average house has 800 to 1,200 square feet. However, most all houses have been added onto by their owners over time. The most common additions have been utility rooms and porches. The developer feels that these additions are a reflection of the greater affluence of the '60s and '70s than existed in the 1950s, when many of the homes were built.

The houses at Orange Gardens were built over a 14-year period (1954-1968). Thus, some houses are over 25 years old. After the initial year of development, 20 houses were built in 1955 and 40 more were built in 1956. After that, about 40 houses were built each year until 1968, when construction stopped. The developer reported that 1968 was the most difficult year for the development of the retirement community. This difficulty was caused by high inflation rates.

Cost to individuals. The initial cost of moving into Orange Gardens consists of the purchase price of the home and lot. In 1955, the cost of homes ranged from $9,000 to $14,000 plus the lot ($900). Prices rose quickly, however, and by 1960 the lots cost $2,000 to $2,500. In 1981, the cost of homes ranged from $30,000 to $45,000. In other words, the prices of homes have tripled or quadrupled since 1955. In addition, one of the 20 vacant lots would now cost about $12,000 (up from $900 in 1955).

There are no monthly charges for living in Orange Gardens. However, residents have the option of joining the Civic Association, which has dues of $2.00 per year.

Demand. There has never been a waiting list to move into Orange Gardens. This is because the developer built houses by order. All houses were custom built.

The demand for houses in Orange Gardens has been reflected in the turnover time for houses being sold. Throughout the history of Orange Gardens, it has not taken long for homes to be sold. In fact, both the developer and the local city planner indicated that the Orange Gardens homes are in the top 25 percent of the homes in Kissimmee with regard to appreciation. This is a reflection of the good quality of the homes and the resulting demand for them. The quality of the homes has also meant low maintenance costs.

There are no plans to continue construction at Orange Gardens. The original development company, Orange Gardens, Inc., has dissolved and the 20 vacant lots are all privately owned. Thus, the only possible future development would be the construction of homes on the vacant lots by the respective owners.

Facilities and Services (F/S)

F/S provided by Orange Gardens. Orange Garden provides a limited assortment of facilities and services. It should be remembered that the strategy of the developer was to build a retirement community near existing services and facilities. In this way, they were available to residents from the beginning of the retirement community and at no cost to the developer.

The major facility provided by Orange Gardens is the Community House, which consists of a meeting room and a library. The Community House was built with money donated by the developer. The developer donated the profits from the first 3 years of sales in Orange Gardens as well as the labor to build the Community House. The Community House is owned and maintained by the Civic Association.

The recreation facilities consist of four shuffleboard courts that are no longer used and are in disrepair. Originally, it was planned to set aside one lot on each block as a recreation or park area. These lots were to be jointly owned by all homeowners of the respective blocks. It was therefore the responsibility of the homeowners to landscape the lots and maintain them as well. In addition, the homeowners were to jointly decide upon specific uses for their block's recreation lot. However, in 1959 (just 5 years after the development of Orange Gardens began), many residents had suggested that the recreation lots had not served their purpose and should be abandoned. Problems had resulted from the lack of families to take on the job of maintaining and managing the lots. Thus, the developer bought the lots back from the Orange Gardens Civic Association, composed of Orange Gardens residents, and built houses on them.

The residents of Orange Gardens also provide a service to themselves. They have formed a "Crime Watch" area in conjunction with the Kissimmee police. In this area, every four houses group together to watch the other three houses in the group. The Orange Gardens "Crime Watch" area has worked so well that the police are now trying to establish similar areas in other parts of town.

F/S provided by surrounding community. The city of Kissimmee provides Orange Gardens with a full range of city services. Police and fire protection are provided by the city as well as refuse collection and all utilities. Kissimmee also has an Art and Culture Center, which includes a civic theater, children's theater, art association, choral group, civic orchestra, historical museum, and a chapter of the Sweet Adelines. Many residents of Orange Gardens are quite active in this center.

F/S provided by private enterprise. Although no shopping facilities exist within Orange Gardens, all of the residents' shopping needs are provided within a one-half mile radius of the retirement community. There is a major grocery store just across the street from Orange Gardens. However, the street is a major four-lane highway through town. Thus, many residents patronize another grocery store a quarter of a mile away so as to not cross the busy street.

The facilities and the services provided at Orange Gardens are summarized in Table 4.1.

Medical Care (MC)

MC provided by Orange Gardens. Orange Gardens provides no medical services or facilities to residents.

MC provided by surrounding area. Kissimmee and Osceola County have an abundant supply of medical services and facilities. There are two hospitals and five nursing homes in Kissimmee. In addition, it is estimated by the developer of Orange Gardens and the city planner that there are about 60 doctors in Osceola County. A home nursing care service is also available in Osceola County. This service provides skilled nursing care (RNs) and home health aides as well as speech and occupational therapy. In order to utilize the home nursing care, a patient must be referred by a physician. Currently, the service has a total of about 49 patients, four of whom are residents of Orange Gardens.

Table 4.2 summarizes the health care facilities and services provided at Orange Gardens.

Ownership/Management/Governance

Type of ownership. Orange Gardens has no single owner. Instead, it is owned by individual homeowners who live there. The developer, Orange Gardens, Inc., is no longer in existence.

Type of management/governance. Orange Gardens is managed by

Table 4.1

PROVIDERS OF FACILITIES AND SERVICES
(NON-MEDICAL)

Location	Retirement Community (Developer/Sponsor/Residents)		Governmental/ Philanthropic	Entrepreneurial
	RC Residents	Non-residents		
Inside RC	community meeting house library shuffleboard courts (4) "Crime Watch" area (by residents)			
Outside RC			fire dept. police arts and culture ctr. refuse collection all utilities	all shopping needs within half mile radius

150

Table 4.2

PROVIDERS OF MEDICAL CARE

Location	Retirement Community (Developer/Sponsor/Residents)		Other Providers (Govt./Philanthropies/Private)
	RC Residents	Non-residents	
Inside RC			
Outside RC			2 hospitals in Kissimmee 5 nursing homes in the Kissimmee area Osceola County home nursing care service About 65 MD's in area

the residents' Civic Association. Membership in the Civic Association is voluntary and costs $2.00 per year. The Civic Association was started in 1955 when about 20 homes had been sold. As a matter of policy, the developer allowed the Civic Association to run Orange Gardens. The purpose of the Association was to involve residents in decisions as to what should or should not be accepted in the community (excluding consideration of individuals). The Association was also responsible for social organizing in the retirement community. However, the Association did not have input into the physical planning of Orange Gardens. Since 1971, when Orange Gardens, Inc. dissolved, the Civic Association has been solely responsible for the rules and regulations of Orange Gardens.

Degree of resident involvement in governance. Even though membership in the Civic Association is voluntary, most all residents belong. The Association has also been an active group throughout the history of Orange Gardens. It was through this group that the "Crime Watch" area was established. The Civic Association also vetoed the development of two small shopping areas in Orange Gardens that had been part of the original plan. The residents decided that they preferred a strictly residential area. It was also through the Civic Association that it was decided to abandon the idea of using one lot per block as a recreational or park lot. Thus, the Civic Association has had a voice in how Orange Gardens was developed and has a reputation throughout Kissimmee as being a vibrant and active force in community affairs.

Financing

Initial costs. The developer of Orange Gardens used $10,000 of his own savings and another $50,000 from investors to begin developing the retirement community. Houses were sold at the cost to the developer plus 20 percent. Of the 20 percent, 15 percent was used to pay commissions, builders, etc., leaving 5 percent for profit. The developer indicated that, in the long run, he made more money selling lots than houses. It is also important to note that the total added cost for the extra safety features included in the houses was only $75 per house. The developer felt this demonstrated that it did not take money to build housing that was responsive to the needs of older people, just awareness of, and attention to, these needs.

Operating costs. The operating costs of Orange Gardens were insignificant because the resident owned their homes and lots and were also responsible for running the community.

Tax structure. All land in Orange Gardens is privately owned and the individual homeowners pay their own property taxes.

Sources of revenue. As stated earlier, the initial source of revenue for the development of Orange Gardens was the developer's own savings and the investment of other individuals. Revenue to continue development came slowly from the sale of homes within the retirement community.

Marketing and Plans for the Future

Advertising. Billboards have been the main form of advertising since the inception of Orange Gardens. In 1956, Orange Gardens began placing billboards all over Florida which resulted in about 200 billboards by 1968. Smaller signs were also placed in Georgia and South Carolina. Easy housekeeping was the main feature stressed in the marketing of Orange Gardens. Safety features included in the homes, such as grab bars, were not stressed. The developer felt safety was not something people wanted to hear about. However, for most residents, safety became an important issue after they moved into the community. Thus, the safety features made the homes responsive to the changing needs of residents as they grew older. This has contributed to the stability of the resident population and to satisfaction with their housing.

Orange Gardens received another form of publicity that was unanticipated. The University of Michigan's Institute of Gerontology made a film about the planning and development of Orange Gardens in 1954. The Institute had been a consultant to the developer during the planning of the community. This film plus the accompanying journal articles were good advertising for the retirement community. The developer reported that, since 1955, responses to the articles have been worldwide. Over 100 inquiries were received per month during the development years.

Future plans. Development of Orange Gardens was completed in 1968 and the development corporation, Orange Gardens, Inc., was dissolved in 1971. The Civic Association now maintains control over the retirement community and is primarily concerned with maintaining its quality.

Overview—Impacts of Change

Effects of change in Orange Gardens. During the period of development, Orange Gardens had a fairly substantial impact on Kissimmee and the surrounding area. Many retirees were attracted to the town because of Orange Gardens, but some chose to move into less expensive housing elsewhere in Kissimmee. This influx of new residents raised the tax base of Kissimmee rapidly while not placing excessively greater demands on public services. For example, there was little or no burden placed on the school system as a result of the development of Orange Gardens. In 1962, when there were 260 homes in Orange Gardens, a local newspaper article discussed the benefits of having Orange Gardens in Kissimmee. It was reported that Orange Gardens residents spent $60,000 monthly, or about three-quarters of a million dollars per year, in Kissimmee. In addition, the homes in Orange Gardens were reported to have added $2,600,000 to the taxable property of Kissimmee. It was also estimated that 5,000 visitors per year came to see Kissimmee and Orange Gardens as a direct result of the road signs and billboards advertising "Orange Gardens in Kissimmee."

Orange Gardens also had an effect on the physical growth of Kissimmee. The major road to Orange Gardens was initially a two-lane dirt road. Soon after the development of Orange Gardens began, the road was paved and widened to four lanes. Initially, no commercial establishments were attracted to the area except a convenience grocery store. Eventually, the road became a major highway and attracted strip commercial development. Today, this highway is a major access route to Disney World and is heavily travelled.

Effects of change in surrounding area. In 1968, the surrounding area had little affect on the development of Orange Gardens. However, recent developments in the area have adversely affected the retirement community. The major four-lane street bounding Orange Gardens provides access to Disney World. Prior to the Disney development in 1971, the highway was lightly used. However, since the opening of Disney World, the traffic and the accompanying noise and pollution have increased greatly, impacting on the houses that adjoin the highway. As a result, these homes have deteriorated compared to the rest of Orange Gardens. The Kissimmee City Planner indicated that the houses along this major street may eventually be bought by the city so as to widen the street. A 50 to 75 foot setback from the road could then be established. The residents of Orange Gardens reportedly favor this plan but would also like the city to construct an eight-foot fence to buffer the highway noise. Clearly, the rapid development of the surrounding area is a concern to the residents of Orange Gardens.

Summary

Orange Gardens was the first subdivision in the country to be architecturally designed for retirement living. However, it was also planned that 15 to 20 percent of the residents should be younger families, some of which would have young children in the household. The homes built in Orange Gardens were designed to accommodate the changing needs of residents by being barrier free, permitting easy maintenance, and including special design features. Orange Gardens was also designed to be assimilated into the surrounding community of Kissimmee. Over the years, this has occurred to such an extent that many townspeople think of Orange Gardens as a high quality subdivision, not a retirement community. In light of this successful assimilation and the acceptance of Orange Gardens housing by people of all ages, the developer has concluded that housing which is good for older people is also good for everyone.

TRAILER ESTATES, MANATEE COUNTY, FLORIDA

General Description

Trailer Estates is a retirement ''subdivision'' with dwelling units composed of mobile homes. Established in 1955, it was the first mobile home development in the country offering the ownership of both mobile homes and lots. The retirement community is owned by its residents and has no medical facilities within it. There are no age restrictions placed on residency.

A plan of Trailer Estates is provided in Figure 4.3.

Location. Trailer Estates is located in an unincorporated area of Manatee County between Bradenton and Sarasota, Florida. It is bounded on the east by a commercial strip (Highway 41), on the south by Sarasota Bay, and on the north and west by subdivisions consisting of single-family homes. These neighboring homes are fairly small and in the $30,000 to $55,000 price range.

Manatee County is the 17th fastest growing county in the country. Currently it is growing at a rate of 4 to 6 percent per year. In 1960, the County's population was about 69,000; in 1970 it was about 97,000; and by 1980, it had reached 145,000.

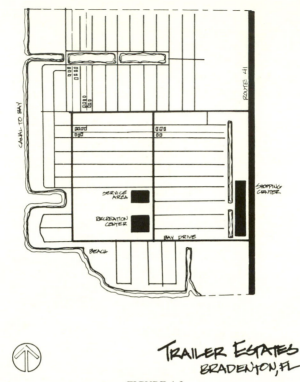

TRAILER ESTATES
BRADENTON, FL

FIGURE 4.3

Manatee County also has a high proportion of older people. In the 1960s the percentage of older people increased dramatically. Only 22 percent of the County's population was over 65 years of age in the 1960s. These population figures remained fairly stable in the '70s. In 1980, the median age of all Manatee County residents was 52 and people over 65 years of age accounted for 31 percent of the total population.

Trailer Estates is located just north of Sarasota County, which is also experiencing rapid growth. According to a planner in the County Planning Department, the County has the highest per capita income in the State and the quality of life and the environment are quite attractive. The Sarasota Standard Metropolitan Statistical Area (SMSA) is the third fastest growing SMSA in the country. Sarasota County also has a high proportion of older people. The figures in Table 4.3 illustrate the County's growth and percentage of older people.

These figures illustrate rapid growth in total population as well as in the percentage of older people.

A regional map showing the location of Trailer Estates is illustrated in Figure 4.4.

Size. Trailer estates is located in a 135-acre tract of land and it

Table 4.3

Sarasota County Population Figures

Year	Population	% Elderly
1960	77,000	18
1970	120,000	29
1980	202,000	35

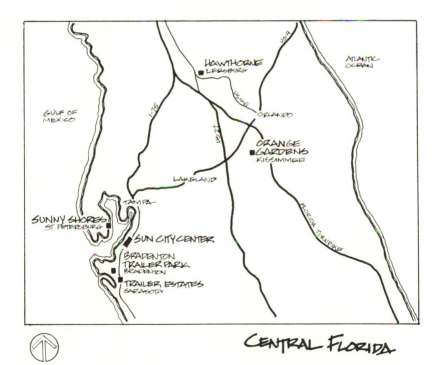

FIGURE 4.4

contains 1,268 mobile homes although it is plotted for 1,500 units. Since some resident buy 1-½ or two lots for their mobile homes, there are fewer units in the park than the maximum possible capacity. However, there are no vacant lots in Trailer Estates. In early 1981, the population was 2,250. During the summer, however, the population is only about half this size due to the large number of seasonal residents.

History.   The development of Trailer Estates was begun in 1955 when the Gulf Development Corporation assembled 125 acres of undeveloped land between Sarasota and Bradenton. Trailer Estates was unique in that mobile home lots were to be sold to the residents instead of rented as in other mobile home developments.

Each purchaser was issued a warranty deed with commitments running until the year 2000. The warranty deed committed the developer to provide the following services for a maintenance fee not to exceed $120 per year per lot: water, sewer service, garbage collection (twice a week), trash pick-up (once a week), TV service, and maintenance of the entire subdivision and all recreation facilities. Thus, the developer was committed to provide these services at no more than $120 per year per lot for the next 45 years. This was a commitment that would later prove problematic.

Lots were initially sold before most of the facilities were constructed. When the first lots were sold, the streets were not blacktopped and the boat basin, auditorium, and 22 of the 32 shuffleboard courts were not constructed. To compensate for this inconvenience, initial residents were not required to pay the full maintenance fee. Despite the lack of facilities, 257 lots were sold in 1955.

Over the next three years, most of the remaining lots were sold and the facilities were completed. By the end of 1959, all but 39 of the 1,433 available lots had been sold and the clubhouse, office building, post office with grocery, and auditorium had been built.[1] Additions were later made to Trailer Estates, raising the total number of lots to 1,500.

By 1971, the developer was having trouble providing services with the $120 per year ceiling placed on payments. Consequently, services to the residents were cut back. This action not only angered residents but also reduced the values of the homes and made them harder to sell by diminishing the attractiveness of the development.

---

[1]The discrepancy between 1,433 available lots and the 1,500 plotted lots is due to some residents keeping one and a-half or two lots for their mobile homes.

As a direct result of the cutback of services, the residents of Trailer Estates began action to purchase the mobile home community themselves. Although the decision to purchase Trailer Estates was not unanimous among residents, most wanted control over the use of monies paid into the maintenance fund. Thus, in 1971, the residents purchased Trailer Estates from the developer for $275,000. A bank loan was needed for the purchase.

To purchase Trailer Estates, residents formed it into a special taxing district named "Trailer Estates Park and Recreation District." This district allowed residents to assess fees against themselves without the approval of another governing body such as the county commissioners. In addition, this action resulted in tax exempt status (state sales and federal income tax) for the retirement community. Thus, by forming a Park and Recreation District, the residents themselves could decide how their assessment income was to be spent and what direction the future development of Trailer Estates would take. Trailer Estates was the first retirement community to follow this course of action. In fact, the state legislature had to write the legislation necessary to make Trailer Estates a Park and Recreation District. Since then, another trailer park in Sarasota (Tri-Par) has also followed this course of action.

By 1972, the residents had elected a representative body with many powers of local units of government, including that of taxation and issuing bonds. In addition, all basic services had been established and all available lots were occupied. The success of resident ownership of Trailer Estates is illustrated by the mobile park's current worth of about $675,000 (September 1980). This is in contrast to a value of $275,000 paid by the residents for Trailer Estates just a little over 10 years ago.

Philosophy

The basic philosophy behind the development of Trailer Estates was to allow residents to purchase not only the mobile home but its lot as well. Early market studies of Trailer Estates revealed that buyers of lots and homes were people from northern and midwestern states who wanted a way to move from a large home to a smaller one. These people wanted to maintain the pride of ownership and have a small piece of property to take care of.

Another benefit of lot ownership concerns financing opportunities. According to Florida tax regulations, if one owns a mobile home and lot, it is considered real property. On the other hand, if only the mobile home is owned, it is considered personal property. This distinction is significant because financial institutions have been reluctant to grant long-term loans for personal property. Thus, by purchasing the lot, residents are able to obtain long-term loans, if needed.

Still another advantage of lot ownership concerns property taxes. In Florida, if one owns property and thus pays property tax then as a Florida resident one is able to take advantage of the Florida Homestead Exemption. The exemption is for $10,000 of assessed value. In addition, the exemption is increased another $5,000 if the person is over 65 years old and has lived in Florida for over 5 years. These exemptions plus a regulation limiting a mobile home's tax evaluation to a maximum of $20,000 mean that some residents pay minimal property taxes per year.

The physical design of the mobile home development is also distinctive. First of all, lots are placed at a 30 degree angle from the street. This configuration provides more privacy and better window views that, in turn, allow high density without making residents feel cramped. Another design concept utilized in Trailer Estates concerned lot size. The developer felt that the prime selling features in a retirement market were opportunities for shared activities and easy maintenance. As a result, individual lots were made smaller and common areas made more extensive than might be designed for a mobile home park housing more children.

Resident Characteristics

Number of residents. As noted earlier, the size of the population of Trailer Estates varies greatly between summer and winter. In the winter months, there are about 2,500 people in the community. However, in the summer months about half of the residents leave to go back to their second homes in the northern states.

Admission requirements. The trailer park is generally an adults-only community with a minimum age for residency of 18. However, families with children under 12 are allowed to live in the park but must live in a specific 3½ block area within the retirement community. Despite the lack of age restrictions, Trailer Estates remains a retirement community by providing services and activities which attract older people—a process of self-selection.

Socioeconomic and demographic profile. In early 1981, the average age of residents was about 70 years. The age distribution of residents was as follows: 30 percent over 75 years of age, 45 percent between 65 and 74 years of age, and 25 percent less than 65 years of age. In recent years, there has been a tendency for new residents to be younger. In 1981, new residents averaged about 61 years of age. This decrease in age was attributed by management to greater numbers of people taking early retirement.

About two-thirds of the households in Trailer Estates are composed of married couples; the remainder are occupied by widows and widowers. There are about 250 to 300 widows living in Trailer Estates. Of the total population, 60 percent are women.

The residents of Trailer Estates are all white and most are Protestant, although religious affiliations vary.

The socioeconomic profile of residents reveals that on the average, they are a middle-to-lower-middle class group of people. This characterization is somewhat misleading, however, since the economic status of residents varies widely. Reportedly, there are very wealthy people living there as well as one person who is on welfare. Former occupations of residents include: teachers, college professors, salespeople, nurses, owners of small businesses, farmers, policemen, firemen, postal workers, lawyers, doctors, dentists, and factory workers and owners. It is truly a diverse group. Most residents are completely retired; only 5 percent work full-time and another 5 percent work part-time. Those who work largely do so in the Bradenton/Sarasota area.

Closely related to their occupational background is the variation in the residents' educational attainment. The average Trailer Estate resident has completed 12 years of formal schooling. About 36 percent have less than 12 years of school; 42 percent have earned a high school degree; 15 percent have had some college training; and 8 percent are college graduates.

The residents are quite active. Although there are no health data on Trailer Estates residents they appear to be a healthy and active group of people.

Residential history. Trailer Estates has a large percentage of seasonal residents. Only half of the residents live there year-round and two-thirds spend at least half the year there.

The residency of Trailer Estates has been very stable as most people tend to stay there permanently once they move in. Residents have lived there 10 years, on the average. A recent survey revealed that 13 percent have lived there since 1954-59, another 28 percent since 1960-70, and 59 percent since 1970-80.

The majority of residents originate from either midwestern or northeastern states. Forty-nine percent moved from the Midwest, 30 percent from the Northeast, 16 percent from Florida and 5 percent from California, Canada, and other southeast states. Florida and Ohio are the most represented states followed by New York, Michigan, Wisconsin, and Indiana. The president of the Board of Trustees reported that almost all of the Florida residents come from outside the Bradenton/Sarasota area.

Trailer Estates residents come from a variety of residential settings and types of housing. Thirty-eight percent of the residents came from urban areas, 28 percent from small towns, 22 percent from suburban areas, and 12 percent from rural areas. In addition, 80 percent of the residents had previously owned a single-family detached home. Only 8 percent lived in a duplex or apartment, 8 percent came from mobile homes, and 3 percent came from farms. However, 29 percent had lived in a mobile home at some time in their lives.

According to a recent survey, there are two major reasons why people move to Trailer Estates. Forty-two percent of the respondents said they moved there because they had friends or relatives already living in Trailer Estates. Twenty-five percent reported that they liked the idea of owning land. Also mentioned were the convenient location (12 percent) and the location on the water (9 percent). It should be noted that of the 117 residents who answered the question, "Do you think there are significant advantages to owning your own land rather than renting?," 114, or 97 percent, replied "yes." This is a clear indication that these residents favor this relatively new ownership arrangement for mobile home developments.

Although most residents remain in Trailer Estates once they move in, some do leave. Those who move away cannot adjust to the high density living of a mobile home park or find it difficult to enter into group activity. Others merely become homesick for their families and move back to their place of origin.

Level of activity. The residents of Trailer Estates are very active within the retirement community. For example, the Shuffleboard Club has 500 members, bingo attracts 475 residents, the Card Club has over 500 people, the beach is used by 100 people per day in the summer, and there are bicycle and yacht clubs as well. A recent study by a local research firm concluded that the Trailer Estates community is more closely knit and active than many communities comprised of the same age groups or Florida residential communities in general. The research firm speculated that this was due to the presence of friends or relatives already in or near the community.

The Trailer Estates residents are also actively involved in the surrounding community. Trailer Estates belongs to the Federation of Manatee County Community Associations for the area mobile home developments. This organization works with the Manatee County Board of Commissioners in the interest of mobile home developments. Residents are also involved with the Gray Ladies in hospitals, boat safety training at the Sarasota Yacht Club, Meals-on-Wheels, and Manatee County services for the elderly.

Trailer Estates is organized as a separate voting district. Traditionally, Trailer Estates residents turn out to vote in higher numbers than residents in other areas of the County. They also tend to vote more conservatively than the surrounding area. In the past, local political candidates have felt that the retirement community vote was important enough to campaign personally there.

Staff. Trailer Estates employs a very small staff. It is composed of an office manager, a maintenance crew of three, one person to care for the meeting hall, and two part-time employees for security and gardening. All other jobs like repairs, etc. are contracted to firms in the surrounding community. Most of the five full-time and two part-time staff members live in the park.

Housing

Size and mix of housing stock. Trailer Estates is composed entirely of mobile homes. In early 1981, there were 1,268 mobile homes in the development. Of these, about 180 are located on waterfront property with direct access to Sarasota Bay.

The mobile homes are about half single-wides and half double-wides with the single-wides generally being older. Single-wide mobile homes in Trailer Estates are generally 8 feet wide and 32 feet long. Their lots are usually 40 by 60 feet and platted at a density of four or five per acre. The double-wide mobile homes are about 1,100 square feet in size plus exterior patios. Mobile homes in Trailer Estates average 750 square feet.

The mobile homes vary as to the number of rooms they contain. About 50 percent have two bedrooms, 40 percent have one bedroom, and 10 percent have three bedrooms. In addition, 75 to 80 percent have a single bathroom while the others have a bath and a half.

Because the mobile homes are not installed at ground level, they are not barrier-free. A tier of three steps is generally required at the entrances of the mobile homes. In addition, the interior doorways are not wide enough to permit passage of a wheelchair.

Mobile homes in Trailer Estates vary greatly in age. About 10 percent of them are about 25 years old and another 15 percent are only 5 years old. Generally, there are more units over 10 years old than under 10 years old. These age statistics may be misleading, however, because about 60 percent of the mobile homes have been modified in some way. Modification may include adding a room, installing new siding, etc. Thus, many older units do not look their age.

Residents of Trailer Estates own their mobile homes and the lots. As stated earlier in the "History" section, Trailer Estates was one of the first mobile home developments in the country to offer residents ownership of the mobile home lot. It is also possible for a mobile home owner to rent his or her unit to another person. In early 1981, about 50 units were being rented, many by young couples. Mobile home owners who rent out their units are usually planning ahead for their retirement. These people can buy a home, rent it for a few years to pay for it, and then retire to it. Although management tries to discourage this practice, it has not legal means to do so.

The developer of Trailer Estates claims that it is advantageous for residents to own their mobile home lots for several reasons. First, residents do not have to worry about rent increases. Second, ownership breeds pride and better upkeep of the development. Third, the residents have control of the park. Thus, there is no tenant/management conflict. Fourth, the mobile home is considered real property if the lot is owned and personal property if the lot is rented. With the real property designation, owners are qualified for long-term financing (20-30 years vs. 15 years). Interest rates on loans for real property are also lower (16 percent vs. 17-18 percent). Still another advantage to owning the mobile home lot is that appreciation is more rapid since real property appreciates faster than personal property.

Costs to individuals. The initial cost of moving into Trailer Estates is the combined purchase price of the mobile home and the lot. In early 1981, these prices ranged from $18,000 to $70,000, with the average being somewhat less than $40,000.

Prices of homes and lots in Trailer Estates have increased a great deal since it opened in 1955. Initially, the developer sold only lots.

A standard lot cost $898 and a corner lot cost $998. Also in 1955, mobile homes with lots sold for $8,000 to $9,000. In 1981, these same units sold for about $30,000—an increase of over 200 percent.

The monthly costs of living in Trailer Estates consist of utility charges and assessment fees. Each resident is responsible for payment of his/her own utilities such as water, electricity, gas, sewer, and telephone. In addition, each household is assessed a $16 monthly fee. The assessment pays for garbage pick-up, maintenance of common areas, street lights, improvement of facilities and recreation areas, and cable TV. Residents pay this fee by adding $180 to their yearly property taxes. Residents are also assessed $15 per year for fire protection which is provided by Trailer Estates' own volunteer fire department and emergency service.

Demand. Since the residents of Trailer Estates own their own homes, no waiting list is maintained. However, the demand for housing is illustrated by the fact that half of the homes for sale are sold before being listed in the open market.

To meet the demand for housing, Trailer Estates is expanding. However, since there is little adjoining land available for development, the expansion is small in scale. The expansion is being made possible by an independent developer who is developing a 3½ acre tract of adjoining land into 21 mobile home lots. After development is completed (1982), this land is to be annexed to Trailer Estates at no cost except the initial cable TV and street lights. Aside from this annexation, there is no further available adjoining land on which to expand.

Facilities and Services (F/S)

F/S provided by Trailer Estates. The services and facilities provided by Trailer Estates are generally recreation oriented. Most of the services are provided in an auditorium complex. In the complex are several rooms for crafts or meetings as well as a large auditorium. Numerous activities are held in the complex, including square dancing, potlucks, ballroom dancing, card games, movies, bingo, and craft/hobby work. Many clubs use the meeting rooms, too. There is a Yacht Club, Grandmothers' Club, Shuffleboard Club, Bicycle Club, and many others. A religious group also holds services in the recreation center. The Trailer Estates Evangelical Covenant Church is a non-denominational church that frequently has over 600 in attendance.

In addition to the recreation complex, there are several outdoor recreation facilities in Trailer Estates. There are 32 shuffleboard courts complete with bleachers for spectators. Since Trailer Estates is situated on Sarasota Bay, it also contains a marina and beach area. About 75 residents have boats in the 150-boat marina. The remaining spaces are rented to non-residents. In early 1981, the monthly rental for boat spaces ranged from $7 to $12 for property owners and $17 to $24 for non-residents. There is even a Trailer Estates Yacht Club which is open to all people who rent spaces in the marina. However, the Yacht Club is largely composed of Trailer Estates residents and there is not much social interaction between the residents and non-residents.

Among the support facilities in Trailer Estates are a post office and a laundromat. The laundromat was needed because residents do not have a washer and dryer in their mobile homes. The post office in Trailer Estates is a contract facility with its own postmaster. Each resident has a post office box since mail is not delivered directly to the homes. Residents consider their post office an important part of their community because it draws people together each day. It has become a central place to see and meet fellow residents and to conduct casual socialization.

Trailer Estates also has its own volunteer fire department. It was started in 1960 when a used fire truck was bought from Fort Blanding, Georgia, for $175. In 1963, the Trailer Estates Fire Control District was created so that a tax base could replace freewill contributions. Then in 1964, a new fire station was built and a new fire truck was purchased. The fire station is manned by volunteers from Trailer Estates who have received training in advanced emergency care.

F/S provided by surrounding community. Trailer Estates is serviced in several ways by Manatee County. The County furnishes police protection through the Sheriff's Office. It also provides water and sewer service although these utilities were originally installed by the developer of Trailer Estates. Bus transportation is also provided by the County which schedules a bus running between Bradenton and Sarasota to stop at Trailer Estates every hour during the day hours. The County provides free transportation to doctors' appointments for low-income people as well. Since Trailer Estates is located between Bradenton and Sarasota and close to Tampa/St. Petersburg, many forms of cultural and entertainment activities are also within close proximity.

F/S provided by private enterprise. There are numerous nearby

shopping and entertainment opportunities provided by the private
sector. Two shopping centers are located very close to Trailer
Estates. One center adjoins it and contains a grocery store, drug
store, cleaners, hardware store, barber shop, furniture shop, bank,
and more. Another larger shopping center is only a half mile away.
Restaurants are also plentiful. Within 5 miles of Trailer Estates
there are 43 restaurants. Residents often schedule bus trips to the
many nearby entertainment attractions. These trips, which are paid
for by the residents themselves, usually include dinner, transportation, and entertainment.

Another service provided by private enterprise is garbage collection. Trailer Estates contracts with a private garbage collection
company as a means to save money. The service costs the retirement
community $4,400 per month. This is roughly 60 percent less than
could be provided by the County.

A summary of the facilities and services provided at Trailer
Estates is provided in Table 4.4.

Medical Care (MC)

MC provided by Trailer Estates. No nursing or medical care is
available in Trailer Estates. However, there is an emergency crew
in the volunteer fire department which can provide assistance in
medical emergencies until County paramedics arrive. The emergency crew is composed of residents who have received training in ad-
vanced emergency care. If a resident needs nursing care, it is the responsibility of the individual and/or his family, not Trailer Estates,
to obtain it. Some residents move to local nursing facilities, but most
move closer to their families in other parts of the County.

MC provided by government/philanthropic organizations. There
are several health-related services and facilities provided by government and/or philanthropic organizations close to Trailer Estates.
Four hospitals are located within 10 miles and a County paramedic
unit is located next to the retirement community. There are also
numerous doctors nearby. One doctor, who has an office just across
the street from Trailer Estates, treats only residents of four local
mobile home parks, including Trailer Estates. He makes house calls
at night and only treats people over 50 years of age.

Manatee County also has a Visiting Nurses Association. This service provides in-home nursing care by RNs and aides to patients

Table 4.4

PROVIDERS OF FACILITIES AND SERVICES
(NON-MEDICAL)

Location	Retirement Community (Developer/Sponsor/Residents)		Governmental/ Philanthropic	Entrepreneurial
	RC Residents	Non-residents		
Inside RC	clubs: bicycle club yacht club grandmother club shuffleboard club shuffleboard courts (32) auditorium square dancing potlucks hobbies card games ballroom dancing church services laundromat marina fire station and protection beach area picnic area		post office police protection utilities (built by developer but bought by county)	garbage collection contracted to private company
Outside RC			free transport-ation to doctor by county transportation to Bradenton and Sarasota by county police protection	shopping centers - one adjoins Trailer Estates - another is 1/2 to 3/4 mile away 43 restaurants within 5 miles of Trailer Estates

recommended by a doctor. This is a valuable service to residents of Trailer Estates and it is used by many of them.

Table 4.5 summarizes the medical services provided at Trailer Estates.

Ownership/Management/Governance

Type of ownership. Trailer Estates is owned by the residents. In 1971, the residents bought the mobile home development from the developer by forming a Park and Recreation District. The formation of a special district was necessary to enable residents to assess fees against themselves without the approval of any other governmental body. These fees are used to operate and maintain the community. The only element of Trailer Estates not owned by the residents is the street system. The streets are owned and maintained by the County. It should be noted that ownership of streets is one difference between subdivision and condominium mobile home developments. Condominium mobile home developments are private property; the residents own and maintain the streets. This allows them to install security gates at entrances to the development if so desired. On the other hand, in subdivision mobile home developments, it is impossible to install security gates since the streets are publicly owned.

Type of management/governance. When Trailer Estates began in 1955, it was run by a manager who was hired by the developer (Gulf Development Corporation). However, management has been a function of the Board of Trustees, composed of residents, since the park became operational as a special taxing district in 1971. Currently, Trailer Estates has neither a manager nor a paid activities director, which saves the residents about $45,000 per year in salary payments. The Board of Trustees consists of nine members who serve without pay. It is required that trustees be residents of Trailer Estates. Management duties are divided among the trustees in the following categories: future planning; recreation activities; treasurer; secretary; maintenance and improvements; grounds; public relations (deed enforcement); and health and welfare (helps obtain services from County).

Degree of resident involvement in governance. The residents of Trailer Estates have a long history of involvement in the governance of the mobile home park. As early as 1955 when Trailer Estates opened, a property owners group was organized to meet with the management "for the betterment of Trailer Estates." In 1957, a

Table 4.5

PROVIDERS OF MEDICAL CARE

Location	Retirement Community (Developer/Sponsor/Residents)		Other Providers (Govt./Philanthropies/Private)
	RC Residents	Non-residents	
Inside RC	emergency crew		
Outside RC			Visiting Nurses Association 4 hospitals County paramedics Nursing homes

nine-member citizens' council was elected by the residents. The Council was then incorporated as the Trailer Estates Property Owner-Resident Association in 1964. This organization had 11 directors composed of residents.

After the residents bought Trailer Estates in 1971, their involvement in governance obviously became more extensive. As stated earlier, the residents began managing the mobile home park themselves in 1971, after deciding not to rehire the previous manager and activities director. To illustrate the extent of resident involvement in the governance of Trailer Estates, the residents donated over 50,000 hours of work in 1979. For example, residents refinished the shuffleboard courts, ran bingo gatherings two nights a week, and did minor plumbing chores throughout the park. The residents feel that managing the park themselves is beneficial because it keeps residents involved in active community life. It also saves them money.

Financing

Initial costs. When originally developing Trailer Estates, the Gulf Development Corporation bought a large tract of undeveloped land. Since Trailer Estates occupied only a portion of the purchased land, it is difficult to determine the original development costs. However, it is known that the residents paid $275,000 when they bought the mobile home park from the developer in 1971. Currently, it is valued at about $675,000.

Operating costs. The costs of operating Trailer Estates are paid and managed by the Board of Trustees. In 1980, the total operating costs were about $242,000, which included payments on the $275,000 loan needed to purchase the park. In addition to these costs, about $50,000 is kept in a contingency fund for emergencies. The total income for 1980 was about $225,000 which mostly came from assessments to the residents.

The trustee meetings and budget operations are open to all Trailer Estates residents. On the average, about 100 residents attend these meetings. In order to ensure that the trustees do not abuse their position, capital expenditures of $10,000 or more cannot be made without a vote of the residents.

Tax structure. Since Trailer Estates has been considered a Park and Recreation District, the common land has been tax exempt. However, the County collects 3 percent of the assessment fees charged to the residents by Trailer Estates (1½ percent for appraiser and 1½ percent for taxes). Residents also pay taxes to the County on their individually owned lots. Florida's Homestead Tax Exemption makes these property tax payments quite low. The tax evaluation of Trailer Estates' mobile homes is a maximum of $20,000 and the Homestead Tax Exemption is for $10,000. In addition, the tax exemption is increased another $5,000 if the person is over 65 years of age and has lived in Florida for over 5 years. Thus, residents pay minimal property taxes.

Sources of revenue. The source of revenue used to originally develop Trailer Estates is unknown. However, the $275,000 paid by the residents to purchase the community was obtained by a bank loan. The day-to-day operations of Trailer Estates is financed by the assessment fees charged to residents.

Marketing and Plans for the Future

Advertising. Trailer Estates does not advertise, not even in the Yellow Pages. Sales are fostered solely by referrals. To assist referrals, a 24-page booklet has been published that serves as a source of information for potential residents.

Future plans. As stated previously in the "Housing" section of this case study, Trailer Estates has little land area on which to expand. Plans call for the annexation of a tract of land with 21 mobile home lots. In light of the limited amount of available land, future plans focus more on improving facilities than adding mobile home lots. Currently, there is interest in installing a swimming pool and whirlpool, although Trailer Estates already provides residents with a private beach in Sarasota Bay.

Overview—Impacts of Change

Effects of change in Trailer Estates. One of the changes that has occurred in Trailer Estates concerns the growth in the number of residents who own their mobile homes. Initially, the mobile homes were sold only to owner occupants. Now, there are about 50 units that are rentals (out of 1,268). The increase in renters began about 10 to 12 years ago and is attributed to an increase in the number of people who choose early retirement. Early retirees have tended to rent instead of buy because they have had smaller pensions and have been too young to receive social security. In addition, some have chosen to rent so as to explore a new life-style. The opposite has also happened in that some people have bought mobile homes in Trailer Estates who are not retired. This change has taken place in the last 10 years or so.

The major effect Trailer Estates has had on the surrounding community concerns the method by which the residents bought it from the developer. Since the Trailer Estates experience represented the first time a Park and Recreation District had been established to facilitate such a purchase, it has since served as a model. For example, the residents of Tri-Par mobile home park in Sarasota have used this same strategy in purchasing that development from its developer.

Effects of change in the surroundings. Most of the changes in the surrounding area that have affected Trailer Estates concern the rapid growth of the area. One such change has been the drastic increase in traffic on U.S. 41, a major highway that adjoins the mobile home park. The traffic has created noise and difficult driving conditions. However, a new branch of I-75, which will by-pass Bradenton and Sarasota, is expected to relieve this situation in 1982.

Another problem created by the surrounding area's growth is caused by the close proximity of the airport. Trailer Estates is located only 1,500 yards from the end of a runway. The residents are bothered by the noise and also fear a crash. As a result, the residents of Trailer Estates would like to see the airport moved away from populated areas. This is a difficult situation because the airport existed before Trailer Estates and most of the surrounding development. However, the advocates for moving the airport point out that the airport was not always as busy as it is now. For example, the airport serviced its first jets in 1961. By 1980, the airport serviced 90 flights a day. This represents a dramatic increase in air traffic that has had a negative impact on the surrounding area.

Summary

Established in 1955, Trailer Estates was the first mobile home development in the country offering the ownership of both mobile homes and lots. The developer, Gulf Development Corporation, saw three advantages to this form of ownership. First, it allowed residents to maintain the pride of ownership and to have a small piece of property to take care of. Second, it meant that the mobile homes were considered real property instead of personal property. Thus, residents would be able to obtain long-term loans, if needed.

Third, residents would be able to take advantage of the Florida Homestead Exemption in the payment of property taxes.

Trailer Estates was also the first retirement community in Florida that was purchased by its residents. In 1971, the residents bought the mobile home park for $275,000. From then on, the residents managed the park and were able to decide how their assessment income was spent and what direction any future development would take. Residents of other mobile home retirement subdivisions have since followed the example of Trailer Estates and purchased their retirement communities too.

Chapter 5

Retirement Residences

BAPTIST GARDENS, LONG BEACH, CALIFORNIA

General Description

Baptist Gardens (BG) is a 13-story "retirement residence" containing 200 one-bedroom apartments plus spaces for social and recreational activities. It was designed for low-income persons 62 years of age and older who are able to live independently. The facility was built in 1975 under the HUD Section 236 Program. It is owned and operated by a non-profit, charitable corporation, sponsored by the First Baptist Church of Long Beach.

A site plan of Baptist Gardens is illustrated in Figure 5.1.

Location. Baptist Gardens is located on the eastern edge of downtown Long Beach, California in Los Angeles County. Long Beach is on the Pacific Coast and was originally a beach town. The mild climate has continued to attract people, especially the elderly, even as the city has developed as a major port.

Between 1900 and 1960 the population of Long Beach steadily grew as a result of residential development and annexation of adjacent developed lands. For the most part, the characteristics of the population have not changed. During this period, the residents consisted of predominantly white, middle-income families. There was also a relatively high (13 percent) percentage of persons 62 years and older.

Since 1960, this situation has been changing. While the rate of growth in the overall population decreased between 1960 and 1980, growth in the non-white sector increased to about 30 percent in 1978. This pattern was characteristic of Los Angeles County. Until recently, the percentage of elderly has remained fairly constant; in 1981, it was estimated at 20 percent of the total population.

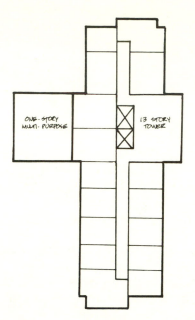

BAPTIST GARDENS
LONG BEACH, CA

FIGURE 5.1

Low-income families and the elderly are concentrated in the downtown area where housing is older and less expensive. This area has deteriorated since 1960 but the elderly choose to live there because of the availability of affordable housing, public transportation, the proximity to governmental services and commercial services, and the quality of air and climate. Traditionally, downtown Long Beach has been a desirable place to live and is considered to be a vital and active neighborhood.

Since the early 1960s, there has been a need for low-cost housing in the downtown area. Little was available. In 1969 the city and local developers responded to this need primarily through the construction of subsidized housing units. By 1981, 5 percent of the housing stock was subsidized and over 60 percent was for the elderly. According to a local housing official, the response was too late and the need is still great.

In 1975, the city adopted a downtown plan for urban renewal.

The immediate impact has been to make the situation for seniors more critical since nearly half of the persons forced to relocate as a result of the renewal program have been senior citizens. The availability of adequate housing lags behind despite the city's requirement that all very low, low, and moderate income units removed be replaced.

In 1981, the City of Long Beach faced a new dimension to the crisis. HUD indicated its reluctance to provide more funding for subsidized housing until the city achieved a more balanced demographic profile. HUD felt the elderly of Long Beach had been over-served and that the city has received more than its share of housing subsidies.

A regional map illustrating the location of Baptist Gardens is shown in Figure 5.2.

Size. Baptist Gardens is a 13-story facility with 200 one-bedroom apartments. Occupancy is restricted to two persons per unit or 400 persons. The population has remained relatively constant at about 225 persons.

History. Baptist Gardens is typical of the housing built in Long Beach in response to the needs of the elderly. It is a subsidized facility located adjacent to downtown Long Beach. The idea for BG began in 1972 when the members of the First Baptist Church of Long Beach recognized the housing needs of the increasing number of low-income elderly in their congregation. A desire to help their own church members led to the formation of Baptist Gardens, Inc., to sponsor the development of the residential facility. The Board of Directors of Baptist Gardens, Inc. contacted consultants who had experience in arranging for the construction and financing of low-cost housing. This group suggested applying to HUD for Section 236 funding because it provides mortgage insurance, interest subsidies, and operating subsidies. Because of the financing, occupancy of Baptist Gardens could not be restricted to Church members. There was an immediate high demand for housing in Baptist Gardens as soon as the plans were announced, reflecting the need that exists in Long Beach.

Philosophy

Baptist Gardens was built to provide low-cost rental housing for the elderly in Long Beach, California. It was designed with facilities and services "to meet the physical, social and psychological needs

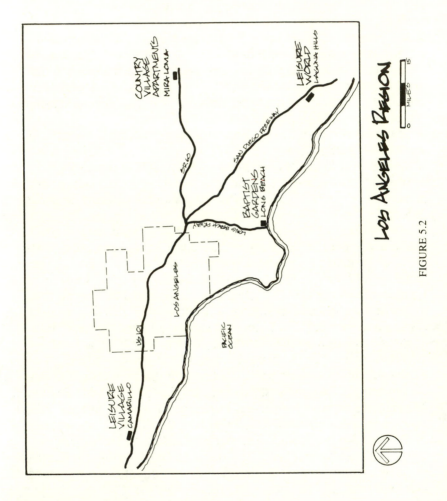

LOS ANGELES REGION

FIGURE 5.2

178

of the aged and contribute to their health, security, happiness and longer living.''

Resident Characteristics

Number of residents. The population of Baptist Gardens has remained about 225 since the facility opened in 1975.

Admission requirements. Occupancy is restricted to persons 62 years old or older and who are able to live independently. Exceptions are made for handicapped people under 62 years of age. Residents sign a Policy Statement agreeing to move from BG when they are no longer able to care for themselves. Preference for occupancy is given to minority and low-income persons and persons displaced by the city's urban renewal program.

Socioeconomic and demographic profile. The population of BG is relatively homogeneous. The average age has increased slightly, from 74 to 76 years, since the facility opened. About half of the residents are between 70 and 80 years old but ages range from 50 to 96.

About three-quarters of residents are single women; no more than 10 percent are married couples. The manager tries to keep a balance between couples and single men and women when considering applications.

Though no data on religious affiliation are available, it has been estimated that the majority of BG residents are Protestants and that 20 percent attend the Baptist Church. The minority population has increased slightly since the facility opened but has never exceeded 5 percent.

Baptist Gardens was designed for persons with low and moderate incomes. The average yearly income of residents is about $6,500; 80 percent of the residents have an annual income of less than $5,500. Many of the residents are former teachers, nurses, and secretaries and are now fully retired. Residents are healthy for their age. They are mentally alert and not frail. The manager described residents as ''vibrant.'' They are able to do their own laundry, shopping, cooking, and to get around on public transportation. Another indication of residents' health is the few calls the city ambulance service receives each month from BG, usually for residents with chest pains, high blood pressure, or mini-strokes.

Residential history. BG is the residents' permanent home. There are no seasonal residents. In 1978, nearly three-quarters had lived in BG since it opened. Yearly turnover has remained less than 10 percent until recently. During the first 6 months of 1981 turnover was more than 10 percent. Nearly all residents lived in Long Beach before moving into BG; a few have come from elsewhere in Los Angeles County.

Many residents move into BG because of a need for low-cost housing and after being displaced by the urban renewal program. The good security and maintenance are also reasons one chooses to live there. Some residents have come to escape the noise and commotion of children, or to escape isolation.

A need for greater health care is the primary reason residents leave BG. Death or a desire to be near family are other reasons residents leave the facility.

Level of activity. The most popular BG activities are the social events. About 40 percent of the residents come to the weekly social hour and a third of the residents regularly attend the pancake breakfast. The monthly birthday parties are also popular. A few residents are extremely active within the facility. They volunteer as lobby sitters to open the door and take calls from residents with a problem. There are two couples that volunteer to be on-call in case of an emergency and one resident writes a column for the BG newsletter. However, residents do not make much use of the recreational facilities available at BG. Most are independent and active outside the facility though the extent of this activity varies.

There are a few residents who play golf or bowl. Another group of residents formed a singing group which performs at convalescent homes, the Senior Citizens' Center, and other places in Long Beach. They have their own band and the money they raise is used for the handicapped. Almost all residents of BG use the Senior Citizen Center. It is a place for social gathering and has services for referral to needed agencies or for volunteer work. Some residents volunteer at the Center. It was established through the efforts of one of the BG residents. Some residents are politically active. They are involved in promoting the rights of the elderly; they attend city council meetings and campaign for candidates. Other residents volunteer at local hospitals or are involved in various church activities. A few are involved in AA and some, 15 to 20, take classes from satellite schools of Long Beach Community College. Many residents spend the day shopping and running errands.

Interpersonal relations between the staff and residents are good, though in 1981 there was a period of getting acquainted after a time of high staff turnover. This was disruptive to many residents and there was both an overall drop in recreational activity and some dissatisfaction expressed to the management company.

Staff. The BG staff is small. There is a manager, tenant-relations/activities director, office assistant, building superintendent, one full-time and one part-time janitor, one full-time and three part-time persons in food service, and a maintenance staff of three. This is a staff-to-resident ratio of about one-to-twenty. One staff member lives in BG while other employees live within 30 miles. All employees are hired by the management company. In the past, turnover was fairly high because of the low pay, but has stabilized recently.

Housing

Size and mix of housing stock. Baptist Gardens is a 13-story residential facility containing 200 one-bedroom rental apartments. Each apartment is 540 square feet and opens onto a balcony. The first residents moved into BG in 1976.

Cost to residents. Residents of BG pay an initial damage deposit and monthly rent which includes all utilities. BG has two rental structures, the Fair Market Rate (FMR) and Basic Rent (BR). Each is based on actual operating costs but FMR is determined on the basis of full interest payments on the mortgage whereas BR is determined on the basis of operating the project with interest-reduction payments which are part of the Section 236 program.

When BG opened the FMR was $295 and the BR was $145; by 1970 the FMR had increased 10 percent to $323 and the BR nearly 20 percent to $170. The greatest increase occurred in 1980 when the FMR went up to $360, an 11 percent increase and the BR increased 23 percent to $210.

The actual rent residents pay, however, varies with their ability to pay. Under Section 236 rent paid is equal to 25 percent of a resident's income or the Basic Rate, whichever is greater, but not exceeding the Fair Market Rate. However, nearly 90 percent of BG residents receive rental assistance.[1] A resident is eligible for rental assistance if 25 percent of his/her income is below the Basic Rent rate.

Under Section 236 no more than 40 percent of the units may be

---

[1]Nearly 90 percent of the units are occupied by residents receiving rent subsidies under the Rental Assistance Payments Program (RAPP); the other 10 percent are receiving subsidies from the Long Beach Authority through the Section 8 Finders-Keepers program known as HAPP (Housing Administration Payments Program).

occupied by persons receiving rent subsidies. In Baptist Gardens, however, more than 40 percent of the units were occupied by residents needing rent subsidies. Some residents were paying up to 30 percent of their income for rent. Thus, the management company requested and received from HUD a waiver of this limit in 1978. The basis for the request was the willingness of the Long Beach Housing Authority to provide the subsidies for BG residents in excess of the 40 percent HUD limit.

Demand. There is a great demand for apartments in BG and there has been since the plans for the project were first announced in 1975. Prospective residents began calling as soon as they heard about it and 60 days after management began taking applications, more than 200 people had applied.

In 1981, 1,026 names were on the waiting list; most were single women. The office receives about five new applications each day and about 20 calls for information.

Facilities and Services (F/S)

F/S provided by Baptist Gardens. Baptist Gardens provides both indoor and outdoor spaces for recreation and socializing. The building has a library/lounge, an activity/craft room, a multi-purpose/dining room, and a laundry room. All are on the ground floor. There are outdoor shuffleboard courts and a rose garden with benches.

The activities director organizes a number of activities for the residents. Every Friday morning there is a social hour with rolls and coffee and each month there is a birthday party. Once or twice a month there are pancake breakfasts and at other times dinners, parties, holiday celebrations, and a yearly luau are organized. The activities director also organizes a yearly mini-swap meet where residents exchange old treasures for new ones, and arranges trips for BG residents, usually with residents of another, similar building, managed by the same company. Movies are available at BG and guest speakers present such topics as consumer awareness, nutrition, self-protection and the use of mace. Classes are also offered at BG with instructors from the surrounding area. At one time Long Beach Community College offered courses but they were cancelled because of insufficient demand. The most popular classes are crafts and physical fitness. Vesper services are offered twice a month and residents have organized a Bible study group. The activities director also publishes a newsletter with a calendar of the month's events and the menu for the month.

Baptist Gardens also provides a meal service. The building was originally built with only a party kitchen, because there were not sufficient funds in the original loan for a commercial kitchen. Since there were numerous restaurants within walking distance, this was not seen as a problem. When the restaurants closed, as the area deteriorated, the owners decided to provide meals at Baptist Gardens. This service operated at a deficit and the owners were unsuccessful in increasing voluntary resident support. Finally, they were confronted with the need either to eliminate the service or make it mandatory. They chose the second option because of their belief in the importance of good nutrition for the elderly, and the likelihood of the need for a meal service increasing as the population aged. Another consideration was the number of residents dependent on the voluntary service. In 1979 under a new, HUD-approved policy they were able to require five meals a month as a condition of residency. The meal program is mandatory only for new residents. When it was first proposed, however, a number of residents complained, fearing they would be forced to spend their money on meals.

Baptist Gardens frees residents of responsibility for cleaning, repairs, plumbing, and electrical work. The maintenance staff will even assist residents in changing of a lightbulb. Painting, trash collection, and gardening are handled by outside contractors.

A number of policies and special features at BG are designed for the security and safety of residents. For instance, the front door is locked at all times. Solicitors are strictly forbidden in the building. There is a speaker system for emergency announcements such as evacuation. Every room and closet has sprinklers in case of fire. Finally, there are railings in each hallway.

F/S provided by governmental/philanthropic organizations. Long Beach provides various city services to BG residents. City police and fire departments serve BG and, according to the manager, are protective of the facility and responsive to calls from the residents. The Housing Authority and Department of Social Services are also available for residents but most choose to use the services of the Senior Citizen Center which provides counseling, referral service, and help in finding volunteer work. Long Beach Community College has organized satellite schools where BG seniors take courses.

The First Baptist Church, located across the street from BG, has an extensive social-recreation program which is open to all BG residents. They also hold vesper services at BG twice a month.

Facilities and services provided by BG are summarized in Table 5.1.

Table 5.1

PROVIDERS OF FACILITIES AND SERVICES
(NON-MEDICAL)

| Location | Retirement Community (Developer/Sponsor/Residents) | | Governmental/ Philanthropic | Entrepreneurial |
	RC Residents	Non-residents		
Inside RC	library-lounge activities-craft rooms multi-purpose dining room laundry room recreation and social programs shuffleboard courts maintenance meals		vespers classes	beauty parlor
Outside RC			city services transportation government agencies utilities fire police	commercial financial

Medical Care (MC)

MC provided by Baptist Gardens. Baptist Gardens has no medical services or facilities and residents are required to leave if they need medical care. The management has created certain services to oversee the welfare of the residents and to respond to emergencies. For instance, there is a resident hall monitor who checks doorslides each morning. If the doorslide has not been pushed to indicate the resident is up, the monitor checks to see if he/she is alright. Each apartment also has an emergency call button which rings if there is a fire or if pulled by the resident. The call rings both in the office and in the apartment of one of two volunteer couples when the office is closed.

MC provided by governmental/philanthropic organizations. There are three hospitals near BG, the closest being two blocks away. The city also has numerous doctors and medical clinics. Those which are close to BG were established many years prior to the construction of the facility. Most residents use their own private physician in the area.

Medical facilities and services provided by BG are summarized in Table 5.2.

Ownership/Management/Governance

Type of ownership. Baptist Gardens is owned by Baptist Gardens, Inc., a non-profit corporation of California sponsored by the First Baptist Church of Long Beach. The corporation was formed for the sole purpose of providing "rental housing and related facilities and services for use and occupancy by elderly persons."

Type of management/governance. HUD has final control over the operation and management of BG for the duration of the insured mortgage. This control protects HUD's interests and guarantees compliance with the requirements of Section 236. The procedures for the operation and management of BG are detailed in the Regulatory Agreement, Management Agreement, and Management Plan.

The Regulatory Agreement, entered into by Baptist Gardens, Inc. and HUD, establishes eligibility requirements; restricts the use of the facility; requires prior HUD approval for changes in the rental rates and reconstruction; and requires rents to be based on operating costs and for the owners to provide maintenance, reserve funds, and management of the property.

Table 5.2

PROVIDERS OF MEDICAL CARE

Location	Retirement Community (Developer/Sponsor/Residents)		Other Providers (Govt./Philanthropies/Private)
	RC Residents	Non-residents	
Inside RC	hall monitors couples on call for emergencies emergency call- buttons in rooms		
Outside RC			hospitals ambulance service doctors clinics

It is the responsibility of the Board of Directors of the Baptist Gardens corporation to see that the operation of BG conforms to these regulations. The Board is composed of an odd number of persons but no fewer than seven. Five of the directors must be members of the First Baptist Church.

The Management Agreement exists between the Board and the management company which is Living Opportunities Management Company (LOMCO). The agreement outlines the areas of responsibility of each. Basically, the Board sets policy, sees that the duties are performed, and approves the budget. The management company is responsible for the day-to-day operation of BG. HUD's Management Plan outlines those duties in detail, specifying, for instance, staff positions, procedures for publicizing, determining tenant eligibility, rent collection, maintenance and a repair schedule, and the requirement of providing social services.

Degree of resident involvement in governance. Residents are not involved in managing BG. They are free to offer suggestions to the manager or to write to HUD. While some residents have exercised these options there is no formal involvement.

Financing

Initial costs. Baptist Gardens was built under the HUD Section 236 program. The initial insured construction loan was $5,760,000, for 40 years at 8½ percent interest. The special features of this program are the HUD insurance, interest subsidy, and the rent subsidies. The interest subsidy is paid by HUD to the lender and allows the sponsor to pay a lower interest rate; in the case of BG the interest is only 1 percent.

Operating costs. Operating costs include payroll, utilities, contracts for services, supplies, taxes, insurance, and financial payments. The total has increased yearly. In fiscal year ending 1977, the first year of operation, the total costs were $349,000 ($145/unit/month) and financial payments accounted for more than 50 percent. By fiscal year ending 1980 the total operating costs had increased by nearly 20 percent to $413,000 ($172/unit/month) and financial payments accounted for slightly more than 40 percent.

Rent increases have been requested on the basis of increased operating costs. The specific areas of increase used to justify the request have been utilities, insurance, maintenance contracts, increases in minimum wage laws, repair costs after warranty expiration, and increased replacement funds.

These operating costs do not include the operation of the meal service which HUD requires be kept as a separate account. This service has operated at a deficit since it was first offered.

Tax structure. During the first 2 years of operation, the annual property taxes were over $7,000. As a result of the passage of Proposition 13, they dropped radically to $2,460 in 1979 and to $1,850 in 1980.

Sources of revenue. Baptist Gardens receives revenue from rent payments on the apartments and from subsidies. There is also income from the laundry and vending machines but it provides less than 1 percent of the total income. Income for the first fiscal year ending 1977 was $346,340; rental assistance accounted for 20 percent of this total. By 1980, the total income had increased by nearly 20 percent to $409,430, a third of this amount came from the rental assistance payments which are part of the Section 236 program and from the Housing Authority program from the City of Long Beach.

Marketing and Plans for the Future

Advertising. Because of the high demand, there has never been a need to market the BG retirement community. The reputation of Baptist Gardens is carried word-of-mouth. Management does have an affirmative action program which led to BG being publicized through minority media, churches, and affirmative action organizations.

Future plans. The owners of BG want to construct another "retirement residence," preferably in the same area.

Overview—Impacts of Change

Effects of change in Baptist Gardens. Since its beginning, the primary change in BG has been the requirement of meal service. This distressed some of the residents. A potential source of problems for residents is high staff turnover. If a major turnover were to occur again, residents would feel a loss of support and security.

Baptist Gardens is only one of the many such facilities in Long Beach. Each alone has little impact on the city but together they represent a large and politically potent population.

Effects of change in surrounding community. The neighborhood around BG has been deteriorating, leading to the closing of many businesses which provided services, such as restaurants. At the same time crime in the immediate environs has increased. Crime is a major concern for BG residents, especially in the unprotected area of the parking lot. Other changes in the City of Long Beach have not directly affected BG except, perhaps, to increase the demand for housing in the facility.

Summary

Baptist Gardens is a "retirement residence" built in Long Beach, California under Section 236 to provide housing for low-income elderly. The need for affordable housing has increased as the city's urban renewal program has displaced many families, especially the elderly.

Baptist Gardens has changed little since it opened in 1976. The average age of the population increased slightly. New residents were required to pay for a minimum number of meals as a condition of residency in order to defray operating costs of the kitchen and ensure continuation of the BG meal service for those residents dependent on it. Also, the management company requested and received from HUD an increase in the percentage of residents allowed to receive rental subsidies to meet the needs of the majority of the residents.

The demand for apartments in BG has remained high. This has contributed to the sponsors' desire to build another retirement residence in the same area.

WILLIAMS MEMORIAL RESIDENCE, NEW YORK, NEW YORK

General Description

The Williams Memorial Residence is a "retirement residence" originally opened in 1964 and moved to its present location in 1969. It consists of one 16-story building that has no health care facilities. Williams Memorial is a non-profit facility owned by the Salvation Army and residency is restricted to people over 55 years of age. A plan of the Williams Residence is illustrated in Figure 5.3.

Location. Williams Memorial is located in Manhattan in New York City. It is on the corner of West End Avenue and 95th Street in a neighborhood known as the West Side. This location provides easy

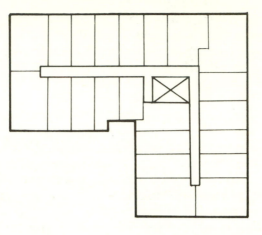

WILLIAMS MEMORIAL
RESIDENCE
NEW YORK, NY

FIGURE 5.3

access to the Lincoln Center, shopping areas, theaters, museums, and other cultural attractions.

New York City is one of the most densely populated and urbanized areas in the world. It is located about equidistant between the metropolitan areas of Boston and Washington, D.C. and is situated at the confluence of the Hudson and East Rivers, with easy access to the Atlantic Ocean. The total area of New York City is about 300 square miles. In 1981 its population was about 7,500,000, resulting in a density of about 26,000 persons per square mile. If daily commuters are added, its population is raised to about 10 million people. Only London and Tokyo can rival these imposing figures.

Manhattan is the oldest and smallest of the five boroughs of New York City. It is 13.4 miles long and only 2.3 miles across at its widest point. Manhattan was once the most populous borough as well. However, since 1950 it has been losing population as homes and apartments make way for commercial and office structures and many people move out to suburban areas. Currently, about 20 percent of the New York City residents (1,500,000) live in Manhattan.

Figure 5.4 shows a regional map with the location of Williams Memorial Residence.

Size. The Williams Memorial Residence is a single 16-story building occupying about a quarter of a city block. Its population in early 1982 was about 430.

History. The building which houses the Residence was originally the Hotel Marcy, a residential hotel built in 1925. In its day, the Hotel Marcy was considered a fashionable residence which over-looked the Hudson River. The Salvation Army purchased the Hotel in 1969 and renamed it the Williams Memorial Residence.

The Salvation Army had maintained a residence for older people in Flushing (located in Queens on Long Island) which was part of a Salvation Army hospital complex. The residence was established in 1964 when money was willed to the Salvation Army for the purpose of providing housing for middle-class older people. Most similar Salvation Army facilities had been funded by HUD, but not the Williams Memorial Residence. Due to the bequest, it has always been a self-supporting facility.

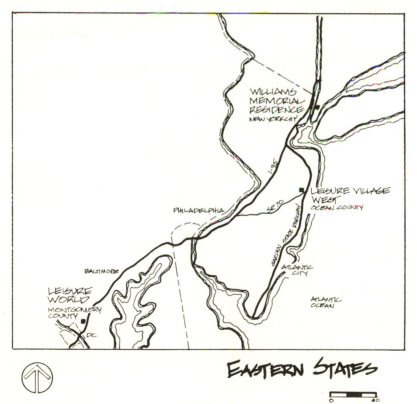

FIGURE 5.4

In the mid-1960s, the Salvation Army hospital needed more space and the Residence was forced to move. Several buildings in the New York City area were considered before deciding on the Hotel Marcy. The Marcy was selected because of its prime location and favorable neighborhood. The Marcy was one block from Broadway and its abundant shopping, and it was relatively close to Lincoln Center. Transportation was readily available since it was on a subway express stop and on a cross town bus connection. The neighborhood was stable and West End Avenue had retained its status and quality. Furthermore, the immediate neighborhood was composed mostly of apartment buildings and an elementary school was located just across the street from the Marcy. Therefore, the neighborhood had a residential character even though it was located in one of the most densely populated areas in the world.

When the Williams Memorial Residence opened in 1969, its first occupants came from two primary places. Some residents moved from the Salvation Army Residence in Flushing which had been closed. Others had been residents of the former Hotel Marcy and remained in the building after the Salvation Army bought it. Within 5 years, the Residence was filled to capacity; almost all residents came from New York City.

Philosophy

Williams Memorial Residence is intended to provide middle-income older men and women with the opportunity of living independently while having access to convenient services. The Residence is operated consistently with the philosophy of the Salvation Army which is an international religious and charitable organization. Officers in the Salvation Army are ordained ministers.

Resident Characteristics

Number of residents. The population of the Residence in early 1982 was 430. The number of residents has remained stable since it reached full capacity in about 1974.

Admission requirements. Criteria for admission to the Residence deal with age, health, and finances. The Residence is open to people of all faiths and residents may also be employed. Residents must be at least 55 years of age to obtain occupancy. In the case of a married couple, only one spouse need be at least 55. The health requirements stipulate that residents must be ambulatory, able to care for themselves, and alert. Financially, the residents must be able to pay the monthly rent. A small percentage of residents receive Supplemental Security Income (SSI), but most are financially independent.

Socioeconomic and demographic profile. The average age of residents has increased in recent years. In early 1982, the average age of residents was about 75 years. A few years ago, it was about 72 years old.

The average age of residents at admission has also increased. In early 1982, it was 76 years with some people being in their 60s and others in their 80s. The Residence would like to reverse this trend and attract younger residents. In order to do so, the minimum age was lowered from 65 to 55 in recent years.

The resident population is largely female. In 1981, 86 percent of the residents were women and there were only eight married couples. Racially, the residents were virtually all white. In early 1982, there were five black elderly living in the Residence. The religious affiliations of residents have changed in the last 5 to 10 years. Six years ago, the residents were about equally divided between Protestants, Catholics, and Jews. Although there may be no causal relationship, the West End of New York City has also become heavily Jewish in recent years. Many of the residents are also first generation immigrants to the U.S.

The socioeconomic profile of residents reveals them to be largely middle-class people. Most had graduated from high school and many were college graduates. Many of the residents had been professionals such as stock brokers and professors. There are also many former housewives living in the Residence. About 10 percent of the residents still work—some for the Residence.

The health of the residents appeared to be pretty good for people of their age (average age approximately 75). Since there is no nursing facility provided, people have to move away when they need nursing care. However, residents are allowed to hire a nursing aide to care for them if such a need arises. This allows people to remain in the Residence after they are no longer able to completely care for themselves. Until recently, residents were not permitted to hire nursing aides. This rule was changed because of the excessive cost of nursing homes and the scarcity of quality nursing homes in the area. In other words, the rule was changed out of concern for the residents.

Residential history. There are no seasonal residents living in the

Residence and about 98 percent remain there until they need nursing care or die. The average length of stay is nearly 9 years. Most residents are from the New York area.

People move into the Residence because of its reputation and location. Most of the residents have lived in New York City for many years and choose Williams Memorial Residence because it is one of the few residences for older people in the city which has nice apartments, relatively low prices, a good location, and which screens it applicants. Many people also move to the Residence because it is owned and operated by the Salvation Army. Residents feel that the Salvation Army is a reputable organization that would operate a high quality and safe facility. Some people move to the Residence because they are afraid of crime in their old neighborhood. Others seek companionship after suffering the loneliness brought on by the death of a spouse. Still others were forced out of their old apartments as a result of condominium or cooperative conversion.

Level of activity. The residents are actively involved in the programs and activities of the Residence. In fact, the administration relies heavily on resident involvement in the organization and operation of many activities. In December 1981, a total of 330 hours of work were volunteered by residents. For example, a retired professor conducted a current events discussion group, a resident dancer teaches a dance class and exercise program, a retired librarian cares for the library, a retired musician teaches music appreciation, and residents operate the gift and snack shop.

Attendance of activities is also heavy. Table 5.3 illustrates the attendance at various types of activities in December of 1981.

Table 5.3
ATTENDANCE OF ACTIVITIES
(December, 1981)

Type of Activity	Number of Events in December	Attendance
Religious Meetings	12	752
Spiritual Development	7	670
Physical Education	2	43
Recreation	18	645
Education	17	274
Social and Special	27	1,562

Resident involvement in the surrounding community is not as extensive as within the Residence. Some residents do volunteer work in the elementary school across the street and in local churches. Many residents also frequent local shops and the museums and theaters in Manhattan. Residents are unlikely to be involved in their old neighborhoods in New York City. This is largely because of changes in the old neighborhood or the problems which led to the decision to move away.

Due to the numerous planned activities in the Residence, there is ample opportunity for residents to interact with the staff. The staff seemed friendly and helpful and their relations with residents seemed pleasant.

Staff. The staff at the Williams Memorial Residence are quite varied because of the wide range of services provided. There are a total of 98 employees in housekeeping, food preparation, maintenance, administration, social service, and health service. The ratio of staff to residents is roughly one-to-four.

The only staff members who live in the Residence are six Salvation Army officers. Other employees live throughout the New York City area.

Housing

Size and mix of housing stock. The Williams Memorial Residence contains 330 apartments in a single 16-story building. The building was built in 1925 and remodeled in 1969 when purchased by the Salvation Army. Residents rent the apartments on a monthly basis.

The Residence offers three types of apartments. There are 24 one-room studio apartments with no kitchenettes, 252 one-room apartments with kitchenettes, and 54 two-room suites with kitchenettes. All apartments are furnished and have private bathrooms and ample closet space. Grab bars and rails have been installed in the tub and shower and handrails are mounted in the hallways of the building.

Costs to individuals. The cost of living at the Residence is the monthly rent. No endowment fees or deposits are required. The following outlines the rent for the various apartments as of early 1982: a single room without a kitchenette ranged from $340-$475 a month; a single room with a kitchenette ranged from $475-$610 a month; and a two-room suite with a kitchenette ranged from $711-$913 a month. Prices for the apartments increase as the floor level increases and include two meals a day, housekeeping services, and all utilities. A small fee is added if a resident has a window air conditioner.

Although rents were held fairly constant for years, they have been increasing sharply in the last few years. Rents increased 8 percent in 1981 and 9 percent in 1980. If a resident were to have difficulty paying the increasing rent, he or she would be advised to apply for Supplemental Security Income (SSI) or move to a lower floor or smaller apartment. This has not occurred as of yet.

Demand. The demand for the apartments in the Williams Memorial Residence varies according to the type of apartment. Two-room suites are the most popular apartments. In early 1982, there were no vacancies in these apartments and a waiting list of prospective residents was being maintained. The one-room apartments without kitchenettes are the least popular apartments. In fact, there are some vacancies among these units. The one-room apartments with kitchenettes are the most common and in the mid-range of demand. There were few, if any, vacancies in these apartments in early 1982.

The demand for various types of apartments has changed over time. The smaller apartments were at one time the most popular. However, as inflation continued and people became more affluent, the larger two-room suites became the most popular. No plans have been made to alter the building so as to provide additional two-room suites because it is felt that the demand for the various apartments is cyclical.

Facilities and Services (F/S)

F/S provided by Williams Memorial Residence. The Williams Memorial Residence provides a wide range of services and facilities. Residents are provided with two meals a day in the cafeteria-style dining room. A third meal may also be purchased à la carte. Between meals, residents may visit the gift shop and snack bar. Recreational facilities include an arts and crafts room, a recreation room with a pool table, and two shuffleboard courts. The Residence also provides a chapel, library, lounge area, and large meeting room. Service facilities include a beauty and barber shop and a laundromat. Residents are also provided with two outdoor patio areas. One is at ground level and the other is on the roof overlooking the Hudson River. The Residence also provides an around-the-clock doorman as a security service.

The activities provided at the Residence are numerous and quite varied as well. In fact, there are generally two or three activities scheduled every day. Religious activities consist of Sunday morning worship services and Tuesday evening vespers. There are spiritual development activities such as Bible classes and related performances. Residents are provided with physical education activities such as exercise classes. Recreational activities consist of movies, craft classes, card games, and dance classes. There are also educational activities such as classes about books, music, and current events. Social and special activities include parties, concerts, and trips to area attractions such as shopping centers, museums, and site-seeing attractions (Bronx Zoo and Brooklyn Botanical Gardens, etc.).

F/S provided by surrounding community. The City of New York contributes the entire range of municipal services to the Residence. Among these services are police and fire protection, utilities, and public transportation including buses and subways. Ample parks are nearby; Central Park is only about 3 blocks to the east and the Hudson River Park is only 2 blocks to the west.

Another service from the surrounding community is volunteerism. Local elementary schools provide frequent choir performances. In addition, students from local colleges frequently perform concerts for the residents. Many of these students come from the nationally known Julliard School of Music which is nearby.

F/S provided by private enterprise. Private enterprise offers the residents minimal services inside the Residence and extensive services outside. Within the Residence, the only service privately provided is the beauty/barber shop. Outside the Residence, shopping and financial services typical of a metropolitan area are readily available. Broadway Avenue is only 1 block away and it is lined with commercial and financial establishments. Grocery stores, drug stores, banks, and restaurants are all within 2 or 3 blocks of the Residence. Taxis are abundant in Manhattan.

F/S provided by the Residence for the surrounding community. The Williams Memorial Residence provides no facilities or services for people of the surrounding community.

A summary of the facilities and services provided at Williams Memorial Residence is provided in Table 5.4.

Table 5.4

PROVIDERS OF FACILITIES AND SERVICES
(NON-MEDICAL)

| Location | Retirement Community (Developer/Sponsor/Residents) | | Governmental/ Philanthropic | Entrepreneurial |
	RC Residents	Non-residents		

Inside RC	roof-top patio
	dining room
	chapel
	library
	lounge area
	large meeting room
	laundromat
	arts & crafts room
	gift shop/snack bar
	recreation room
	ground level patio
	shuffleboard courts (2)
	security door
	telephone in room
	weekly maid service,
	  bedding, linen, and
	  towels
	religious meetings
	spiritual development
	  activities
	physical education
	recreational activities
	a van to take trips
	social events
				beauty and
				barber shops

Outside RC			all municipal
			services by
			N.Y. City
			Central Park
			3 blks away
			buses, subways
			performances by
			music students
			(elem. &
			Juilliard)
				Broadway Ave. 1 blk.
				away has most
				shopping needs --
				  grocery
				  drug store
				  bank
				  restaurants
				  taxis

Medical Care (MC)

MC provided by Williams Memorial Residence. The Residence has no infirmary or nursing care service. However, one registered nurse is on staff and available for emergencies. The nurse works every day until 11:00 p.m. Two physicians have office hours in the Residence each week as well. In addition, the switchboard operator has had practical nurse training and two residents are retired nurses.

If a resident becomes ill, the staff nurse works in cooperation with the resident's physician. Residents may use any physician they choose. In the case of serious illness, nursing home or hospital care are required. The staff social worker helps residents make these arrangements although the resident is responsible for all hospital charges and ambulance or transportation charges. Residents are also responsible for physician's fees, medication, and other aids prescribed by the physician.

MC provided by governmental/philanthropic organizations. All of the medical facilities expected in a large metropolitan area are provided in New York City. St. Luke's Hospital is located about 20 blocks away and there are numerous nursing homes in the New York City area.

MC provided by private enterprise. A variety of private medical services are provided to residents of Williams Memorial. The Residence is affiliated with a private ambulance service to assure prompt emergency response. In addition, some residents hire private nursing aides to live them. This allows the resident to postpone the necessity of moving to a nursing home or some other more medically supported setting. Private physicians also treat the patients as needed.

A summary of the health care facilities provided in Williams Memorial Residence is provided in Table 5.5.

MC provided by the Residence for the surrounding community. The Williams Memorial Residence provides no medical or nursing services to the surrounding community.

Ownership/Management/Governance

Type of ownership. The Residence is a not-for-profit facility owned and operated by the Salvation Army, a religious, charitable, non-profit organization. Salvation Army officers are ordained ministers.

Table 5.5

PROVIDERS OF MEDICAL CARE

Location	Retirement Community (Developer/Sponsor/Residents)		Other Providers (Govt./Philanthropies/Private)
	RC Residents	Non-residents	
Inside RC	staff nurse 2 MD's with office hours		
Outside RC			hospital 20 blocks away affiliation with ambulance service private physicians

Type of Management. The Salvation Army appoints one of its officers to be the administrator of the Residence. The administrator is also assisted by five other Salvation Army officers in this management function.

Degree of Resident involvement in governance. Residents have no role in the governance of the facility or in policy making. In case of problems or complaints, residents go to the staff social worker who attempts to resolve the problem with the administrator. This procedure has evolved because the residents know the social worker well and feel comfortable with her. She has been on staff since the Residence opened in 1969. She knows all of the residents, since admissions are made through her office.

Financing

Initial costs. The Salvation Army paid $1,550,000 for the Hotel Marcy in 1969. Another $650,000 was then spent on renovations in the building.

Operating costs. The total operating costs for the Residence in 1981 were $2,198,000. Of this total, $2,100,000 was budgeted for room and board. Other major budget items were $54,000 for payment of indebtedness (from initial purchase of Residence), and $21,000 for a third meal per day for residents (monthly rental only pays for two meals a day).

Tax structure. Since the Salvation Army is a charitable organization, the Residence is tax exempt.

Sources of revenue. The initial resources to establish the Williams Memorial Residence came from a bequest to the Salvation Army. This money was to be used to establish a residence for middle-class older people. The Salvation Army used the bequest and an additional bank loan to purchase the Hotel Marcy in 1969.

The sole source of revenue for the operation of the Residence is the rental fee charged to residents. Rental rates are fixed so that income will meet operating expenses. Even staff salaries are paid out of rental fees. Self-sufficiency is essential because the Salvation Army supplies no funds for the operation of the Residence.

Marketing and Plans for the Future

Advertising. The Williams Memorial Residence has no advertising campaign. Word-of-mouth and an occasional ad in the New

York Times are the only way prospective residents learn of the Residence.

Future plans. There are currently no plans to expand or remodel the Residence. The goal is to maintain the quality of the facility.

Overview—Impacts of Change

Effects of change in the Residence. It is quite possible that the Williams Memorial Residence has been a positive and stabilizing force in its neighborhood. Since the Salvation Army renovated the Hotel Marcy, there has been much renovation in the immediate neighborhood. Two buildings within 1 block of the Residence are being renovated to house rather costly condominiums. A new apartment building is also being built 1 block away.

Effect of change in surroundings. The Williams Memorial Residence is on the fringe of a large area of New York City undergoing rejuvenation. The boundaries of the area are generally considered to be between 96th Street and 59th Street on New York's West Side. The Residence is located on 95th Street. Even within this general area of rejuvenation, some of the nearby streets are not considered safe for residents to walk at night. Despite the changes occurring around it, the Williams Memorial Residence does not seem to have been affected. On the contrary, the Residence has probably affected the immediate neighborhood more than the neighborhood has affected it. More importantly, the Residence's impact seems to have been quite positive.

Summary

The Williams Memorial Residence has undergone limited change since it opened at its present location in 1969. It has always attracted most all of its residents from the New York City Metropolitan Area and enjoyed a reputation as one of the best residences for middle-class older people in the city. One of the few changes that have occurred concerns residents who become in need of nursing care. Since the Residence provides no nursing facility and there had been a rule forbidding residents from hiring their own nursing aides, residents had to move away when they became in need of nursing care. However, this rule was recently changed to allow residents to hire nursing aides at their own expense. This allows people to remain in the Residence after they are no longer able to completely care for themselves. This change demonstrates a certain amount of adaptability on the part of the Residence in that rules were altered so as to consider the changing needs of residents.

Chapter 6

Continuing Care Retirement Centers

FRIENDSHIP VILLAGE, SCHAUMBURG, ILLINOIS

General Description

Friendship Village is a "continuing care" retirement center. Established in early 1977, it is a non-profit privately owned retirement community housed under one roof. The building is composed of 4 pavilions or semi-detached units. It offers residents extensive health care facilities and services as well as passive indoor recreation/leisure services. Residency is restricted to those at least 52 years old. A plan of Friendship Village is illustrated in Figure 6.1.

Location. Friendship Village is located in Schaumburg, Illinois, a northwestern suburb of Chicago. It is the only continuing care housing development in the Chicago area that features independent, apartment living. For the most part, Friendship Village is surrounded by moderately sized houses built in the late 1960s.

Schaumburg was selected as the site of Friendship Village for two major reasons. First, it was a rapidly growing community which attracts middle-aged executives who may in turn want to be close to their retired parents. Thus, Schaumburg would be a likely place for these parents to live. Second, Schaumburg is also close to O'Hare Airport and Chicago itself. The convenience of a large international airport and shopping and cultural events close by makes Schaumburg very attractive.

The population of Schaumburg grew by 180 percent between 1970 and 1980. In 1970 its population was about 18,500 and by 1980 it had increased to 52,000. During this same period, the number of housing units in Schaumburg increased by about 400 percent. In 1970, there were about 5,000 housing units and by 1980, there were over 20,000.

Schaumburg's growth from 1970 to 1980 was not an isolated phenomenon. The latest census figures show that the population of the western suburban area of the Chicago Metropolitan Area doubled in size from 1970 to 1980.

A regional map showing the location of Friendship Village is illustrated in Figure 6.2.

Size. The Friendship Village complex is situated on 34 acres. The population in 1980 was approximately 900; 767 residents were liv-

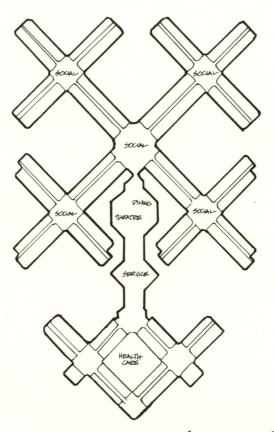

FIGURE 6.1

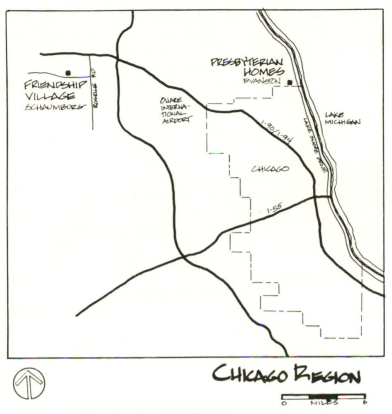

FRIENDSHIP VILLAGE SCHAUMBURG

PRESBYTERIAN HOMES EVANSTON

ROSELLE RD

OHARE INTERNA- TIONAL AIRPORT

I-90/I-94

LAKE SHORE DRIVE

LAKE MICHIGAN

CHICAGO

I-55

CHICAGO REGION

0 MILES 6

FIGURE 6.2

ing in 632 independent units and 122 patients were occupying the 180 beds in the health care unit.

History. Friendship Village was the first non-denominational continuing care facility in the State of Illinois. It opened in two stages: the first in January of 1977 and the second in 1978.

Friendship Village was originally established by the Evangelical Retirement Homes of Greater Chicago, Inc. in 1975. This organization was formed by a group of area ministers and businessmen in cooperation with, and under the direction of, Life Care Services Corporation (LCSC) of Des Moines, Iowa. LCSC is a business that organizes and establishes non-profit organizations to operate retirement communities across the country. However, in 1980, Friendship Village Schaumburg severed its relationship with LCSC and became an independent life-care facility.

In light of the retirement community's past ties to LCSC, a brief history of LCSC is in order. Its history begins with Dr. Kenneth Berg, who has been referred to as the grandfather of the life-care contract concept and the creation of retirement community operations under this concept throughout the U.S. Dr. Berg felt that such retirement communities could be built independent of the church. In the past, this type of retirement community had predominantly been developed under church sponsorship. Between 1965 and 1979, he developed 62 life-care retirement communities in the U.S., mostly in the Midwest. They were all named John Knox Village and were intended for low-income people who did not need Medicaid.

Dr. Berg contracted with one construction company to build all of the John Knox Villages in the country. The contract was awarded to Fred Weitz, President of Weitz Construction Company of Des Moines, Iowa. Eventually, Weitz separated from Berg because he saw problems with the economics of Berg's operation. Upon separation, Weitz formed the Life Care Services Corporation (LCSC). LCSC had direct or indirect involvement in the development of about 20 retirement communities each named Friendship Village. As stated above, Friendship Village of Schaumburg was originally one of these LCSC developments.

Philosophy

The philosophy of Friendship Village is based on the life-care concept. It provides for the comprehensive care of a person from the early, independent retirement years through the period of total dependency.

Comprehensive care at Friendship Village is intended to serve all needs of the residents. The spiritual, social, and physical needs of individuals are provided for in a non-sectarian, inter-faith atmosphere. By providing quality living accommodations and comprehensive health care services, the well-being of the residents is felt to be enhanced and the period of independence and dignity extended.

Friendship Village is intended to serve financially and physically independent elderly adults. It offers a self-determined life-style in a private apartment. Residents are expected to bring their own furniture and personal possessions. The community is designed to attract people who are independent and capable of handling their own affairs but who want the security of knowing that someone is always there if help is needed.

Resident Characteristics

Number of residents. The population of Friendship Village has remained fairly stable throughout its short history. In early 1981, there were about 900 residents. Of these, about 770 lived in independent-living apartments. The remainder lived in the health care unit which has a 180-patient capacity.

The population has remained stable because nearly 80 percent of the first two pavilions were sold before the construction had been completed. Likewise, nearly 50 percent of the second two pavilions were sold prior to their completion. Thus, Friendship Village has enjoyed a near-capacity population since it opened in 1977.

Admission requirements. Three factors are considered in the admissions application for Friendship Village: age, health status, and financial situation. Residents must be at least 52 years old and must also be ambulatory and in good health. Good health is defined as being able to care for oneself for at least 6 months after moving into the facility. Certification of prospective residents' health is obtained within Friendship Village's own health center.

The financial requirements for admission stipulate that a person must have liquid assets and a monthly income sufficient to pay the monthly fee. A "rule of thumb" used to assess a prospective resident's financial acceptability is that he or she must have a net worth of at least twice as much as the initial entrance fee. The fees for residency are discussed in the "Housing" section of this case study. To verify their assets, potential residents must provide a 5-year record of their income tax return.

Friendship Village has a recommendations committee to deal with admissions. The committee is composed of three people: the vice president of the board of directors; the comptroller of the management team; and a specially trained registered nurse. This committee has existed for only 2 years. According to the administrators, admissions were too lax before the committee's inception; too many people were accepted who needed medical care too soon.

Socioeconomic and demographic profile. The average age of residents has increased since Friendship Village opened 4 years ago. In early 1981, the average age of men living in independent housing was 79 and that of women was 78. Four years ago, the average age of residents was about 76.

The average age of people who are admitted has also increased. In early 1981, new residents (both men and women) were 75 years old. In 1977, the average age at admission was 76. The executive director of Friendship Village attributes the increase in the age of new residents to the increased independence of the public in general which allows people to continue living at home for longer periods of time.

The socioeconomic profile of residents reveals that they had largely held white collar professional jobs or were housewives. Residents who lived in Friendship Village in the period from 1977 to 1980 had assets worth, on the average, $390,000. Their average monthly income was about $950. Finally, about one-half to three-fourths of the residents owned cars.

Other available data indicate little change in the population of Friendship Village. The ratio of women to men is about three to one (583 women and 184 men). Thus, the population is largely composed of widowed women. In 1981, there were approximately 110 couples in the facility. The residents are virtually all white and have a broad range of religious backgrounds. The most prominent religions among the resident population are Lutheran, Baptist, Methodist, Catholic, and Presbyterian. Finally, several residents still work. None work full-time but about one-fourth of all residents work part-time in the Chicago area.

For the most part, residents in the independent housing units were healthy and active for their age. Residents housed in the health care unit, on the other hand, were not active. The ratio of independent units to health care units is about four-to-one and, therefore, the healthier, more active residents are most characteristic of the community.

Residential history. Since Friendship Village is so new, very few residents have moved away. Most will remain in the facility until they die. In the 4 years since Friendship Village opened, an average of one person has moved out every 6 months. It has been reported that those who chose to leave were unable to adjust to the new lifestyle and were consequently unhappy.

Friendship Village has few seasonal residents. Virtually everyone lives there throughout the year.

About 90 percent of the Friendship Village residents had previously lived in the Chicago area. In addition, a few long-time Chicago residents who had previously retired to the Sunbelt, have returned to the Chicago area and to Friendship Village. These moves were prompted by their anticipation of failing health.

People move to Friendship Village because of their concern for security and its location. Two types of security are being sought by residents: medical and financial. Medical security takes the form of the health care unit while the financial security occurs through the residents' knowledge that a serious illness will not deplete them or their families of their financial resources. In short, security is provided by the life-care contract offered by Friendship Village.

The location of Friendship Village also attracts people. Because of its proximity to Chicago and the city's cultural amenities and its being within a half-hour from O'Hare Airport, this retirement community is considered a desirable place to live.

Level of activity. The residents of Friendship Village are heavily involved in the activities within their community. These activities, for the most part, are passive in nature, such as reading, playing cards and other games, and participating in arts and crafts.

The Women's Council is one organization arranging activities for residents. It was organized in 1979 and all women living in Friendship Village are members. Monthly meetings are held 10 months out of the year and are attended by roughly 200 women. The Women's Council sponsors a bazaar each year to sell items made by residents. People from the surrounding area attend this bazaar in large numbers. Traffic generated by the bazaar has become so heavy that the local Boy Scouts direct traffic in the parking lot. In the first 3 years of the bazaar, it has made $5,000, $9,500, and $8,500 respectively. The revenues generated from the bazaar have been used to open a gift shop in Friendship Village. After the first 5 months of the gift shop's existence, it was accepted by Dunn and Bradstreet which requires a $10,000 account at all times for a credit rating. The Women's Council has also bought two kilns for the arts and crafts department, five microphones, curtains for the windows of the assembly hall, and various pieces of furniture.

Resident involvement outside the retirement community is not as active as inside. However, many residents like to walk, a few hike, and there are many golfers and bowlers. Neither golf nor bowling is provided within Friendship Village. Although the township offers several services for elderly people, such as free income tax service and legal advice, the residents of Friendship Village do not use them much because they have their own similar services in the retirement community. However, the assistant to the senior citizen coordinator for the township is a resident of Friendship Village. She helps the coordinator organize activities and programs for the elderly who live in the township.

One area of heavy resident involvement in the outside community is voting. Friendship Village is a voting precinct in itself and the residents, who are predominantly Republican, have a history of high voter turnout.

In light of the heavy involvement of the residents within Friendship Village, they have frequent interaction with staff. Informal conversations with residents revealed a friendly and caring relationship between residents and staff. This relationship is evidenced by the residents' Christmas Fund Committee. The residents have formed a committee to collect money from their ranks to be given to employees at Christmas. Last year, over $17,000 was collected and distributed to the staff.

Staff. Because of the wide range of health care and other services provided, over 300 individuals are employed at Friendship Village on either a full-time or part-time basis. These personnel represent a full-time equivalent of 200 staff members. Employees provide the following categories of services: social service, spiritual service, health care services, administration, and miscellaneous support services. None live in Friendship Village but reside throughout the Chicago suburbs.

Housing

Size and mix of housing stock. Friendship Village has all of its independent housing units and its health care units in a single building. There are 632 independent living units and 180 beds in the health care wing of the building. The building is designed as a complex of six pavilions. Independent housing units are located in four of the pavilions which are each 3 stories tall. The health care unit is located in the remaining two pavilions which are each 1 story tall. All of the units are relatively new in that the building was opened as two phases in 1977 and 1978.

The independent living units are available in four sizes. The smallest are the 87 studio apartments. Alcoves are the next largest apartment units and there are 225 of them. Finally, there are 224 one-bedroom apartments and 96 two-bedroom apartments. All apartments are air-conditioned and have full kitchens.

The health care unit has 180 beds in two sizes of rooms: private and semi-private. There are 20 private rooms and 160 semi-private rooms. All the rooms are air-conditioned and have bathrooms.

The payment plan at Friendship Village calls for the resident and the facility to enter into a life-care contract. Residents are required to pay an initial endowment fee plus a monthly fee. The Life-Care Contract offered by Friendship Village does not limit the amount by which the monthly fee may be increased after a person has moved in. Thus, the monthly fee may increase at whatever rate is needed to meet the rising costs of providing services.

Costs to individuals. The initial cost to residents is in the form of an Endowment Fee. In 1981, this endowment fee ranged from about $24,000 to $54,000, depending on the size of the apartment and the number of people who occupy it. The fee is not refunded to a resident's estate upon death. However, a portion of it may be returned to the resident who leaves Friendship Village within 22 months of moving in. If one moves out within this 22-month period, either all but 22 percent of the endowment fee is returned or 1 percent per month until the endowment is depleted is returned, whichever is greater.

A history of the endowment fee reveals that it has not been increasing as rapidly as the country's rate of inflation. In 1979 and 1980, the country's rate of inflation was approximately 27 percent. During those same 2 years, Friendship Village increased the amount of the endowment fee only 16 percent. However, the fee was increased by 14 percent in 1981. In 1977, the endowment fee varied from $18,500 to $44,000. By 1980, it had increased to a range of $23,000 to $51,000. In 1981, the fee varied from $24,000 to $53,500, which represents a 24 percent increase since 1977.

The monthly fee paid by residents has also been increasing over the 4 years of Friendship Village's existence. As noted earlier, there is no limit as to the amount the monthly fee may be increased. The executive director feels strongly that a life-care contract should not contain a limit on the allowable increase in the monthly fee. Limitation in times of high inflation could threaten the economic stability of the facility.

In 1977, the monthly fee ranged from $250 to $400 depending on the type of unit. By 1980, fees had increased to a range of about $375 to $550. In 1981, the fee ranged from about $425 to $625, which represents a 45 percent increase over a 4-year period.

The cost of living in the health care facility is higher than that of the apartments. For residents of Friendship Village, the cost is roughly $115 a month more than the monthly fee. This supplemental charge covers two extra daily meals. In the health center, three daily meals are provided. It should be noted that a resident living alone who needs full-time nursing care must relinquish his or her apartment. If he or she is married, the spouse may stay on. For patients who are not residents of Friendship Village the cost is figured on a daily basis. In early 1981, the cost was $45 a day for skilled nursing care beds and $41 a day for intermediate care beds.

Friendship Village also has a benevolent policy concerning the monthly fee. Even though every effort is made to assure that a prospective resident will be able to afford monthly charges for apartment and health care services, Friendship Village will not evict anyone who can no longer afford the monthly fee.

Demand. The independent housing units of Friendship Village have been fully occupied since shortly after the community opened in 1977. About 80 percent of the first two pavilions were sold prior to their opening and about 50 percent of the second two pavilions were sold before they opened.

Friendship Village currently maintains a waiting list of prospective residents. In early 1981, there were about 40 names on the list. Admission is based on the length of time one's name is on the list, and one's preference for time of admission, location in the complex, and a particular room.

The demand for different types of apartments has changed over time. Originally, the two-bedroom apartment was the most popular. In 1981, the one-bedroom apartment had the longest waiting list. The executive director feels that this change is largely a result of changes in the economy and the unwillingness or inability of people to pay for the two-bedroom apartment. In 1981, there was an 8 month to 12 month wait for a one-bedroom apartment and about a 9 month wait for a two-bedroom apartment. The wait for an alcove or studio apartment was 4 to 6 months. Friendship Village has no plans to build any additional units to meet this demand.

Facilities and Services (F/S)

F/S provided by Friendship Village. Friendship Village has a wide range of services and facilities that make it possible for residents to conduct their lives without having to leave the building. The community has a dining room which serves one hot meal a day, a library, an assembly hall, a room for church services, a convenience food store, large sitting and meeting areas, numerous game areas, an arts and crafts room, and a daily news sheet to inform residents of daily events. In addition, residents receive bi-monthly maid service, weekly flat laundry service, local phone services, and all utilities such as electric, water, gas, and telephone.

The activities director indicated that there is not an abundance of planned activities for the residents. This policy is designed to encourage the residents to plan activities for themselves.

The arts and crafts room provides a place for residents to indulge in woodworking, crafts, pottery, etc. Although 20 percent of the residents already participate in the arts and crafts program, the activities director is seeking to attract more. To do so, it is being proposed that the arts and crafts become decentralized by having several smaller craft rooms located throughout the facility. In this way, the arts and crafts could become more visible and accessible and thus attract more people.

Two services available at Friendship Village are provided by the residents themselves. One is a gift shop and the other is the men's workshop. The men's workshop is operated by residents who fix televisions and other appliances belonging to fellow residents. The service is free.

Church services at Friendship Village are held on Tuesday night. Services are not held on Sunday so residents can attend their own churches elsewhere in the Chicago area. Friendship Village even provides bus transportation to local churches on Sunday. The services at Friendship Village are non-denominational and are attended by a third to a half of the residents. Residents have their own church choir.

Security at Friendship Village includes security guards and the use of video cameras. Guards are hired to patrol the grounds and buildings. The men are not uniformed and are fairly unobtrusive. Each entrance to the building is monitored by a video camera which allows those working at the main entrance to see all who enter.

Friendship Village also owns a small bus. It is used to take residents on trips to local shopping centers as well as to church services.

As shown in Figure 6.1, the design of Friendship Village allows for the intermittent placement of atriums and cozy lounge areas. The atriums are generally large, 3-story tall spaces where informal gathering is common. Adjacent to the atriums are several smaller lounge areas where small groups of residents may sit and talk in relative privacy. Also adjacent to the atriums are alcoves containing pool tables. Informal conversations with residents revealed that they are seldom in their rooms. Instead, they spend time in the atrium and lounge areas where they can meet with friends. In the partially enclosed outdoor areas formed by the pavilions, shuffleboard courts have been installed. As of the spring of 1981, they have not received much use.

Another type of service provided by Friendship Village is life insurance for residents. The policy is offered at a 50 percent discounted rate which is made possible by a group insurance plan. The plan is optional, but will be mandatory within 1 year. Illinois is the first state to offer this insurance plan and Friendship Village is the first retirement community in Illinois to use it.

F/S provided by surrounding community. Individuals and organizations from throughout the surrounding community provide residents of Friendship Village with a seemingly constant flow of entertainment. According to the activities director, too many outside groups are offering their services to Friendship Village and its residents. Local schools provide choirs, bands, and theatrical performances for the residents. Local churches have also sent choir groups. Such activities usually take place in the assembly hall.

A local church group also offers a personal shopper service to Friendship Village residents who are unable to use buses. Church volunteers come to Friendship Village to learn what residents need and then shop for them.

Various city services are available to Friendship Village. Police and fire protection, refuse collection, and bus service are provided by Schaumburg. A city library is also close to Friendship Village.

Schaumburg Township offers other services to the elderly as well. It provides free income tax service and free legal advice for all elderly living in the township. Even though the township offices are 1 block away, few Friendship Village residents utilize these services because they are provided within Friendship Village.

F/S provided by private enterprise. Many privately provided services are available to residents both inside and outside the grounds of Friendship Village. Within Friendship Village, there is a beauty shop and barber shop. A local bank also has a branch office inside the building complex. Finally, there is a travel agent in Friendship Village. Group tours are arranged for residents to various places around the country. For example, a resident group recently visited Williamsburg, Virginia.

Numerous nearby shopping areas are also available to Friendship Village residents. A major shopping mall is located about a mile away. Although it is too far away for most residents to walk, both the city bus service and Friendship Village provide regular transportation.

F/S provided by Friendship Village for the surrounding community. Friendship Village is beginning to offer services for people living outside the retirement community. The activities director indicated that because there are so many services and forms of entertainment for the residents, many of them have become self-centered or inwardly oriented. In an effort to overcome this, the activities director is emphasizing service projects for other groups. For example, a band composed of residents has been sent to a home for retarded children. Other residents have taught English to refugees from Vietnam, Cambodia, and Laos who are brought to Friendship Village. These types of activities have proven to be very rewarding to the residents.

A summary of facilities and services provided at Friendship Village is included in Table 6.1.

Medical Care (MC)

MC provided by Friendship Village. Health care is an important facet of life at Friendship Village as it is in other life-care facilities. The Friendship Village health care center is licensed as a skilled nursing facility. The entire facility is staffed as if it were skilled care even though three levels of care are provided: skilled nursing, intermediate care, and sheltered care. This is a rare arrangement, but the Director of Nursing feels that it is good for patients as well as the nursing staff because it results in a higher staff-to-patient ratio and a higher percentage of RNs on staff than would otherwise be the case. However, it is expensive.

The health care center accepts patients from the outside community if space is available and the patients are able to cover their daily cost. However, priority is given to residents of Friendship Village. This means that patients from outside the community may be evicted if the beds are needed to care for residents of Friendship Village. This has not happened yet. In fact, only 122 of the 180 beds were occupied as of early 1981. Of these, 22 were occupied by temporary care patients who were residents, 24 were occupied by outsiders, and 62 were occupied by life-care patients.

The health care center is divided into two pavilions. One pavilion houses patients with high care needs; the other houses those patients considered confused. Each pavilion has its own dining room. Thus, one dining room is used by patients who are relatively independent and the other is for patients who are totally dependent. Patients are also allowed to eat in the main dining room as long as they sign out

Table 6.1

PROVIDERS OF FACILITIES AND SERVICES
(NON-MEDICAL)

| Location | Retirement Community (Developer/Sponsor/Residents) | | Governmental/ Philanthropic | Entrepreneurial |
	RC Residents	Non-residents		
Inside RC	shuffleboard assembly hall lawyer 7-11 type store arts and crafts bus church services life insurance large atrium area library security guards and cameras food		bus local schools, etc., come to RC to entertain residents Personal Shopper Service	beauty and barber shop bank tours
Outside RC		resident band for retarded children help refugees learn to speak English	fire police	shopping center (10 minutes away)

of the health care center so as to relieve the nursing unit of responsibility.

Sheltered care is provided both in the health care facility and in the independent living units. If a resident of an apartment needs help bathing or dressing but does not need 24-hour nursing care, there are three employees to provide help as needed. The price of this care is included in the monthly fee for the apartment. In early 1981, there were about 30 residents utilizing this service.

The health care facility and its staff offer residents a wide range of medical services. Friendship Village has five part-time physicians. One physician is on 24-hour call. Consulting physicians include a psychiatrist, dentist, podiatrist, urologist, neurologist, opthomologist, and a dermatologist. Physicians are available 3 days a week during set hours. Various independent laboratories also have agreements to visit Friendship Village on a regular basis. These services include occupational therapy, physical therapy, and pharmacy. It should be noted that, if interested, residents are allowed to use their own private doctors, but at their own expense.

The health care unit has its own activities department. Activities in the health care unit are more passive than in the independent housing portion of the facility, but they have a varied and structured program. In addition to the typical reality orientation program, the patients are taken on trips and treated with music therapy. Music therapy is even supplied to patients who are comatose. Patients are taken on trips in the local area about once per week. Trips include going out to lunch, seeing a movie, or visiting places like a museum, zoo, O'Hare Airport, the Chicago Post Office, or going on a picnic.

Friendship Village apartments have several health-related features. Each apartment is furnished with an emergency pull cord. When a resident signals an emergency, one nurse runs to the apartment while another calls the resident on the telephone. The entire health center staff is available for emergency calls from apartments. Each apartment is also furnished with a token to hang on the outside of the front door every night. The tokens are taken in every morning to signal that all is well. Every morning, a staff member walks the halls checking for tokens that are not taken in. If one is found, the person knocks on the door to check if there is a problem. Finally, decals are placed on the exterior of the front door of any resident's apartment who might need help evacuating the building in case of a fire or other emergency. These decals inform firemen and others that the person in that apartment needs help.

The dining room is also equipped with a computerized system that allows the recording of who eats what meal. The system is called a computerized personal accounting system. With the system, it is possible to determine if all residents who were to eat that meal did, in fact, come to the dining room. If the resident was unexpectedly absent, a call is made to the resident's apartment to make sure there is no problem.

There has been one important change in the operation of the health care unit since it opened about 4 years ago. The change concerned admission to the facility. Initially incoming residents were allowed to move directly to the health care unit. This means that people endowed medical rooms just as they would an apartment. This practice was recently discontinued (1979) because there was not enough room to continue it and priority was given the residents of the independent living units. Before this practice ended, eight people had endowed medical rooms. As of early 1981, only three of these people were still alive. The patient care coordinator indicated that the initial policy of allowing new residents to endow health care rooms was an attempt to increase occupancy after Friendship Village first opened.

MC provided by surrounding area. Since Friendship Village provides such a complete health care facility, medical services outside the community are rarely needed, with the exception of the hospitals. Ample hospital facilities are available; there are three within a 10-mile radius.

Table 6.2 summarizes the medical services available at Friendship Village.

Ownership/Management/Governance

Friendship Village is a privately owned, non-profit organization. It has a 12 member Board of Directors made up of local businessmen and clergy of various denominations. The Board was created by LCSC and is now a self-perpetuating Board. To manage Friendship Village, the Board hires an executive director. The executive director is the chief executive officer and is ultimately responsible for the direction, coordination, and overall management of the facility.

Degree of resident involvement in governance. Residents have a voice in the management of Friendship Village through a Resident

Table 6.2

PROVIDERS OF MEDICAL CARE

| Location | Retirement Community (Developer/Sponsor/Residents) | | Other Providers (Govt./Philanthropies/Private) |
	RC Residents	Non-residents	
Inside RC	dining room computer door signs (am) door decals (fire) emergency pull cords in apartments doctor skilled care intermediate care sheltered care dining rooms activities department	nursing care	
Outside RC			three area hospitals ambulance service

Council. The stated purposes of the Resident Council are three-fold:

1. To develop procedures for the residents to participate in decision-making with the administration on matters directly affecting the physical, medical, and general well-being of the residents;
2. To provide a means of dispensing information to residents; and
3. To motivate residents to become active in the Resident Council's operations.

Although the Council has no official governing power, the administration is responsive to it. One way in which the administration involves residents in the operations of Friendship Village is by offering a full financial report to residents quarterly. Residents are permitted to have their personal attorneys inspect the records if they choose. With this information, residents can satisfy themselves that prices actually do have to be increased or that the facility is being operated efficiently. This policy seems to have resulted in a trusting relationship between residents and administration.

The Council is composed of 13 residents who operate under a committee structure. Residents use these committees to voice complaints or suggestions about related concerns.

The Resident Council has been an active organization in the past. One of its major accomplishments was the installation of a traffic light at the entrance to Friendship Village. The street from which to enter Friendship Village is five lanes wide and carries a considerable amount of traffic. Thus, it was difficult for residents with cars and guests to merge into the mainstream of traffic without a traffic light. In an effort to have a light installed, the Resident Council invited state and county representatives to visit Friendship Village. However, the residents were told that it would be at least 2 years before a light could be installed. Unwilling to accept the delay, the residents wrote about 200 letters to state legislators and local government officials. Within 1 year from the initial request, a light had been installed.

Residents are also active in the many issues that confront senior citizens. Action taken by the Council is handled in much the same manner as the traffic light incident.

It is interesting to note that the Resident Council was not originally planned as a vehicle for involving residents in governance of Friendship Village. Instead, it began as a result of a roof cave-in in the dining room in 1979. To help organize the resulting changes in the daily routine of residents, one resident from each of the four pavilions was selected to form a committee. The committee was to help inform and organize the residents during the peirod of roof repair. However, after the dining room was repaired, the residents decided to continue the council and made it an ongoing organization.

Financing

Initial costs. The Prudential Life Insurance Company of America carries the mortgage and obtained the initial funding for Friendship Village. The mortgage is for $13.1 million. The executive director estimated that if Friendship Village were built in early 1981, the cost would be about 40 percent higher because of inflation.

Operating costs. Friendship Village has computed the operating expense for an average apartment per month. This figure is then compared to the operating income for an average apartment to help determine monthly fees. In 1981, the average operating expense per apartment was $10,280, whereas the average operating income was $10,200. The balance of these two figures was taken from the endowment fees. To illustrate how quickly expenses are rising, in 1980 the average operating expense per apartment was $8,750, whereas the average operating income was $9,475.

Tax structure. Friendship Village pays property taxes to Cook County. In the past, they have been about $250,000 per year.

Sources of revenue. The sources of revenue for Friendship Village are three-fold: monthly fees, endowment fees, and the initial mortgage obtained to build the facility.

Marketing and Plans for the Future

Advertising. Although the largest source of advertising for Friendship Village is word-of-mouth, it does have an advertising campaign. Even before it opened in 1977, $2 million was spent to market Friendship Village. Advertising has been focused within the Chicago Metropolitan Area.

Recently, a survey was conducted to determine how people who inquire about living in Friendship Village heard about it. It was found that a friend's referral was the most common source. The second and third most common sources were newspaper ads and current residents, respectively. Thus, out of the three most common sources, two involved word-of-mouth.

Other forms of advertising used by Friendship Village are quite varied. Advertisements have been placed in magazines such as *Christianity Today* and the *Chamber of Commerce Magazine* for the Schaumburg area. The local telephone directory and other surburban directories have also been used, as well as radio commercials. Friendship Village sometimes also allows prospective residents to spend a night in the building to see how they like it. However, this is only possible if there is a vacant apartment.

Future plans. Although there are no formal plans for additional construction, both the executive director and the patient care coordinator voiced a need for additional building to be used for sheltered care. The new facility would be for residents who can no longer live in independent housing, but have no serious medical problem. The patient care coordinator stated that such a facility would not have to be staffed by nurses, but by companions. The companions could have a nursing supervisor to call in cases of emergency.

The patient care coordinator also felt that a "holding area" is needed. Such an area would be used for under 24-hour admission to the health care area such as overnight supervision.

Overview—Impacts of Change

Due to Friendship Village's short history, no major changes in its environs have occurred. Informal conversations with the city planner, city assessor, and others in Schaumburg revealed that Friendship Village is generally considered to have been a positive addition to the community. The residents of Schaumburg seem to be pleased that Friendship Village is attracting a group of people they feel are positive additions to their city.

Summary

Friendship Village is a relatively new "continuing-care" retirement center, having been opened in 1977. It was the first non-denominational continuing-care facility in the State of Illinois. Another factor which distinguishes it from other continuing care facilities we visited is that it is housed in a single building. However, this has not affected other features of the retirement community.

OTTERBEIN HOME,
WARREN COUNTY, OHIO

General Description

Otterbein Home is a "continuing care" retirement community offering extensive health care facilities and passive recreation/leisure activities. It operates as a non-profit organization affiliated with the West Ohio Conference of the United Methodist Church.

Originally begun in 1913, Otterbein Home, herein referred to as Otterbein, now provides three types of independent housing and three levels of health care facilities for its residents. Independent housing units are situated in ranch style duplex apartments, cottages, and newly remodeled apartment buildings. The three levels of health care are personal, intermediate, and skilled nursing.[1] Admission to the independent housing units is restricted to persons 62 years of age or older while applicants for the health care units must be at least 65.

Otterbein is accredited by the Joint Commission on Accreditation of Hospitals and Long-Term Nursing Facilities, and certified by the Health and Welfare Certification Council of the United Methodist Church. In March of 1979, Otterbein was selected as the "Agency of the Year" by the Division of Health and Welfare Ministries, United Methodist Church.

A plan of Otterbein is shown in Figure 6.3.

Location. Otterbein is located in rural Warren County, Ohio, about midway between Dayton and Cincinnati. Lebanon, a town of 9,500, is 3 miles away. Otterbein's complex of buildings is flanked by the Warren County Council On Aging facility, a large private park, the Lebanon Correctional Facility, and Otterbein's own farm land.

Despite its rural character, Warren County is one of the fastest growing counties in Ohio. Growth is attributable to the increasing numbers of people moving from Cincinnati and Dayton. In 1980, 62 percent of Warren County's labor force worked in the adjoining counties.

A regional map illustrating the location of Otterbein is illustrated in Figure 6.4.

Size. In 1980 Otterbein had a population of about 540 residents,

---

[1]See "Medical Care" section for definitions of the three levels of health care.

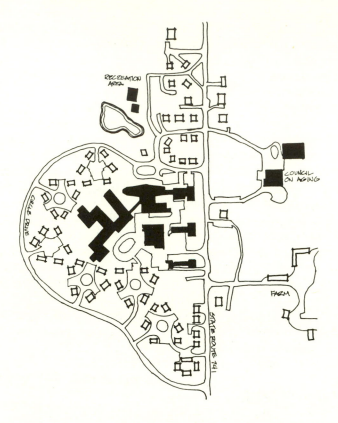

OTTERBEIN HOME
LEBANON, OH

FIGURE 6.3

making it the largest non-profit comprehensive retirement community in Ohio. Otterbein owns about 1,500 acres of land but less
than 100 acres are currently developed. The remaining land is used
for agricultural purposes.

History. Otterbein was founded in 1913 when the United Brethren
Church purchased 4,000 acres from the Shakers, a communal religious sect. The land had been the site of the Shaker Union Village
which was founded in 1805.

Otterbein has evolved through two distinctly different periods and
is presently entering a new third phase of development. In the first

period lasting about 50 years, Otterbein housed children as well as older people and was characterized as a poor farm for the church. The second phase of development began in the mid-1960s. This phase can be described as one of planned growth and improving quality of care that has continued to the present day. The third phase is currently in the planning stage. During the next decade, the Otterbein Master Plan proposes two additional campuses which could roughly triple the size of the present population.

The first phase of Otterbein's history extended from its inception in 1913 to the mid-1960s. During this time, Otterbein was a combination Home for the Aging and Children's Home. Until about 1960, it was viewed as the church's poor farm and subsisted mainly on contributions from the church and from other gifts. During the depression, Otterbein faced economic hardship and consequently sold about half of its land (2,000 acres) to the state. In the late 1950s, the

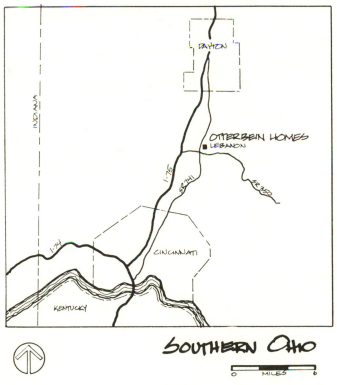

FIGURE 6.4

possibility existed that a Cincinnati-Dayton metropolitan airport would be built nearby in Warren County. This potentiality resulted in a period of no growth because Otterbein's sponsors feared that the airport would be incompatible with the pastoral setting of the retirement community. In 1946, the United Brethren Church (the original sponsor) and the Evangelical Association united to form the Evangelical United Brethren Church.

During the late 1960s, Otterbein underwent a number of changes which, for purposes of this analysis, mark a changeover from the initial phase of development to the second phase. Changes involved the population makeup, the administration, the sponsorship, and the method by which residents paid for housing and other services.

In 1963 the child care program, in operation since Otterbein's inception, was eliminated. It was felt that children would be better served through foster care. The remaining children were placed in a home which specialized in the needs of children. The second change concerned the administration or management. From the mid-1950s to the late 1960s, administrative problems coupled with the uncertainty about the proposed regional airport contributed to extensive physical deterioration. Many of the older buildings did not meet modern codes and, as a result, the State of Ohio threatened to rescind Otterbein's nursing home license. Furthermore, Otterbein was not able to operate economically for the 140 persons who were living there in the mid-1960s.

The third change involved another change in church sponsorship. In 1968, the Evangelical United Brethren Church united with the Methodist Church to become the United Methodist Church. Unlike the previous union, this had a direct impact on the income Otterbein was receiving from its sponsor. Under the Evangelical United Brethren Church, the supporting area of the Midwest region contributed about $200,000 per year to the Home. Under the sponsorship of the United Methodist Church, Otterbein was related to the West Ohio Conference, representing a much smaller geographic area. Consequently, the financial contribution to the support of Otterbein was dramatically reduced to less than $90,000 annually. This represented a reduction of more than 50 percent.

A fourth change concerned the method by which residents paid for housing and other services. Previously, people applying for residency at Otterbein were required to surrender all their financial assets. In the late 1960s, this financial arrangement of payment was abandoned and a straight monthly payment system was initiated.[2] This was supplemented by a refundable life use fee program to help with the construction of new facilities. This change in the method of payment has resulted in a change in Otterbein's image; rather than being viewed as an institution providing custodial care, Otterbein is now considered a community for retirement living serving the elderly with varying financial resources.

In response to the many problems facing Otterbein, a long range planning committee was established in 1967 by the Board of Trustees. The Committee was immediately faced with the decision as to whether Otterbein should expand, move its program to another location, or close its doors. After extensive study, the Committee recommended to the Board of Trustees that Otterbein remain at its present location and expand its facilities on the adjacent land. The expansion aimed at providing additional nursing facilities and housing units devoted to independent housing. A 10-year $9 million expansion program was initiated in the early 1970s; by 1980, the population had increased to more than 500 people, existing buildings had been remodeled, and new central service and nursing buildings and 84 duplex units had been built.

The 1980s constitute the third stage of Otterbein's development. The Master Plan proposes two additional campuses, each of which would house approximately 500 residents. A total population could reach 1,500 to 1,800.

Philosophy

The stated purpose of Otterbein is to provide a supportive environment that enables elderly residents in various stages of physical and emotional need to live meaningful and satisfying lives in as independent a manner as possible. Otterbein strives to encourage the maximum amount of possible self-help and mutual-help among residents. By helping themselves and their neighbors, residents act as providers of support and assistance and not merely as consumers. The intent is to encourage the maximum involvement of residents in all phases of living. A by-product of the policy of self-help and mutual assistance is reduction in costs; total reliance

---

[2]The refundable life use fee is discussed in detail under "Housing."

on the staff to perform supportive functions is discouraged. Thus, the need for a large staff is minimized.

Resident Characteristics

In 1970, the population of Otterbein was 187 with a capacity of 214 residents. During the 1970s, there had been a total of 900 people residing at Otterbein. Approximately 40 percent lived in independent housing and the remainder occupied the health care units.

Number of residents. In 1981, there were about 540 residents in Otterbein with a maximum capacity of 670. The difference between the population and capacity is attributable to the fact that many two-person dwelling units were occupied by only one person. As of spring 1981, Otterbein had no vacant units. Otterbein has grown since it became strictly a retirement community in the mid-1960s, when it housed about 140 residents.

Admissions requirements. Admission to Otterbein is restricted according to age and, to a lesser extent, place of residence and financial resources. Persons 62 years of age or older are eligible for residence in the independent living units, while persons aged 65 or older are eligible for the health care areas. If a couple has applied, only one is required to meet the age requirement. Mentally or physically handicapped persons aged 40 or older may also be admitted if they are accompanied by a parent who is at least 62 years old. Applications are accepted from "well" ambulatory persons seeking facilities for retirement living as well as from persons who need nursing care.

In April 1981, there were 1,800 names on an admissions waiting list. While length of time on the list is an important consideration in selecting residents, geographic, financial, and religious considerations also enter into the selection procedure. Priority is given to the applicants living within the jurisdiction of the West Ohio Conference of the United Methodist Church. For example, although prospective residents need not be United Methodist to be accepted, no United Methodist Church member and no resident of Butler, Montgomery, and Warren Counties of Ohio (needing health care) is refused admission because of a lack of funds. Priority may also be given to the United Methodist missionaries, ministers, minister's widows, and lay-church employees of the West Ohio Conference.

Socioeconomic and demographic profile. The average age of

residents at Otterbein has increased slightly over the last 10 years. In 1981 the average age of all residents was 82.5 years, whereas in 1970 it was 80.5 years. For women there was virtually no change, whereas for men the average age increased substantially. In 1970 the typical male resident was slightly over 76; in 1980 he was 82. Over the past 4 years, four-fifths of the population has been women. This proportion has remained fairly constant over the last 10 years.

People living in independent housing were younger than residents of the health care areas. Independent housing residents averaged 78 years while people in the health care units were 85 years old on the average. In 1980, the average age at entry was about 79 years; admissions to the health care units averaged 82 years old and those entering the independent housing averaged about 77 years old.

Other available data indicate that the types of residents have not dramatically changed over the last 10 years. Two-thirds of the residents were employed in professional, managerial, or business occupations. The remaining one-third worked in clerical, domestic, or farm-related activities. The education of the average resident has been gradually increasing as more professional persons move to Otterbein. About 40 percent of the residents own their own cars. The residents were almost exclusively white and more than 8 in 10 admitted during the last 11 years were United Methodists. Finally, virtually all residents were fully retired and permanent residents of Otterbein.

The health of Otterbein residents manifests itself in the types of housing units people occupy. In 1980, there were 211 people living in the independent housing and 327 living in the health care units. During the last 4 years, the number of independent housing residents has decreased slightly (6 percent). At the same time, the number of residents occupying health care units has increased by 8 percent.

An examination of the changes in the health of residents and their average age reveals an interesting pattern. Despite the fact that more people who lived in independent housing have moved to Otterbein during the last 10 years, the average age of residents has remained at about 82 years. It would appear, therefore, that the addition of independent housing units has not attracted the young elderly. This is evidenced by the fact that the average age of those living in independent housing was 78 years in 1980. Therefore, despite changes in the size of the total population and the housing types offered, Otterbein has, for the most part, remained a retirement community for the old elderly who seek the security offered by the health care facilities.

Residential history. The length of time that people reside at Otterbein varies depending on the degree of health care they need. The average length of residence for persons living in independent housing was 7 years. Residents lived in the personal care units for an average of 5 years. And lastly, residents of the skilled nursing area resided at Otterbein only 2 years. These differences reflect life expectancies rather than decisions to move away.

Most Otterbein residents previously lived in the surrounding area; 60 percent lived within a 30-mile radius and 70 percent had a rural background. Over the past decade the market area has decreased in size because of the increase in the numbers and quality of housing and nursing facilities for the elderly built elsewhere in Ohio and changes in church conference relations.

Surprisingly, about 10 percent of the residents moved to Otterbein from Florida or other Sunbelt states. Many of them had originally lived in Ohio. One explanation for the return was the security offered by the health care facilities at Otterbein.

Similarities also exist among the residents with respect to their former housing. Seventy-eight percent owned and occupied private homes and 15 percent came from nursing homes. Only 6 percent moved to Otterbein from hospitals and less than 1 percent were mental hospital patients.

Interviews with the administrative staff revealed several reasons why people moved to Otterbein. The two most frequently mentioned explanations were the security offered by the health care facilities and Otterbein's affiliation with the United Methodist Church. The church affiliation was important and for many residents, the presence of a church on the premises was a source of great pride. Other reasons for moving to Otterbein were its attractive rural setting and its non-institutional character. In fact, administrative efforts were made to create a "home-like" atmosphere. Still another attraction is the familiarity and past experience applicants have had with Otterbein; a number of children of former residents have applied for admission in recent years.

Few people have moved from Otterbein; most remain until their death. Among those who do leave, two factors influence their decision. First, according to staff members, some people have difficulty severing ties with the past and choose to return to their former homes. Others find cheaper care elsewhere and move because of difficulties affording rising costs.

Level of activity. An inventory of the interests among residents prepared by staff revealed a high preference for passive pursuits. Activities of greatest interest were reading, gardening, music, travel, cards and other games, needlework, and knitting. Activities with low levels of interest were active pursuits such as bowling, bicycling, dancing, golf, and swimming.

A number of Otterbein residents are active outside the immediate community and interact with area residents. Social events are held at Otterbein which attract people from Lebanon and other nearby towns. For example, a youth conference is held each year, during which time high school students from Lebanon come to Otterbein and participate in a day of discussion and interchange.

Another form of social interaction outside of Otterbein is provided by the Geronteers, a volunteer group from the surrounding area who work in Otterbein. They perform needed services such as shopping for residents, helping to feed residents, pushing wheel chairs, giving manicures, and mending clothing.

Otterbein also provides its residents with transportation to and from Lebanon twice a week as well as numerous daily trips for medical appointments off campus. Several residents also drive their own cars to Lebanon or other nearby towns for shopping and social purposes. A few of the residents also make use of the YMCA in Lebanon and the senior citizen center across the street from the home.

Staff. In 1981, the staff at Otterbein consisted of about 370 employees, resulting in a staff-to-patient ratio of 2-to-3. The types of employees are quite varied because of the wide range of health care and other services provided. Categories of salaried personnel include social services (social workers and activity directors), spiritual services (clergy), health care services (doctors and nurses), and various support staff. Personnel are discussed in more detail in the "Medical" and the "Services" sections of this case study. The volunteer staff consists of a group called the Geronteers (see earlier mention) and resident volunteers.

Relationships between the staff and patients reflect the supportive nature of Otterbein. Staff members are encouraged to interact with residents and offer assistance whenever possible. This is intended to create a friendly home atmosphere which will foster a sense of belonging among residents. In conversations with residents, several of them mentioned how much they liked and appreciated the friendly and helpful staff.

Housing

Size and character of housing stock. Otterbein provides both independent housing units and health care units. There are 176 units categorized as independent housing and 356 beds in three levels of health care.

Otterbein has been planned with the idea that 300 to 500 residents is the optimal size for a retirement community. A population of less than 200 is considered uneconomical in light of the level of services provided. By comparison, populations over 500 are viewed as too large for residents and staff to know and recognize each other.

The physical layout for the retirement community reflects this small scale philosophy while the housing units are designed with flexibility in mind. The issue of scale has been addressed in various ways. First, new buildings with congregate housing were designed with hallway breaks or bends so as to minimize their perceived length and to create identifiable sections or neighborhoods within the buildings. Second, small congregate dining rooms accommodating residents during three time-shifts per meal were provided. In this way, residents are able to eat in smaller, more intimate areas. Finally, the independent duplexes have been clustered around cul-de-sac streets so as to foster a sense of neighborhood among their residents.

The issue of flexible housing units is addressed by designing them in a manner that allows two small apartment units to be joined to create one larger apartment. Generally, the smaller units are used for dependent living and the larger units for independent living. Thus, the design and construction of the buildings allows Otterbein to provide facilities which are in current demand by making minor and inexpensive modifications.

Mobility is also encouraged by the physical design of the community in that enclosed walkways connect all resident buildings except the ranch style duplex apartments and cottages. This makes it easier in bad weather for people to venture out of their living quarters. It also encourages interaction among residents needing different levels of care.

Housing mix. Included in the 171 independent units are the congregate buildings, the ranch style duplex apartments, and the cottages. There are two 3-story buildings, Bethany Hall and Phillippi Hall, that contain 62 congregate independent housing units. Bethany Hall has 31 one- and two-room apartments with fully equipped kitchenettes. Phillippi Halls has 30 one-, two- and three-room apartments with kitchenettes and four single rooms. The usual occupancy in the two buildings is 1.33 persons per unit.

Eighty-four ranch style duplex apartments are arranged around cul-de-sacs on the perimeter of the development. Cul-de-sacs have either 12 or 14 apartments, including studio, one-bedroom, and two sizes of the two-bedroom units. Usual occupancy in the duplexes is 1.35 persons per unit.

The third type of independent housing unit is the cottage. In 1981, there were 30 cottages, all of which were built prior to 1960. Thirteen were occupied by employees while the remaining 17 housed residents.

In 1981, construction began on six clusters containing three buildings with a total of 108 apartments. Each of these 1-story buildings contains six apartments with attached garages. A laundromat is provided for each cluster.

All independent housing units are barrier free except some of the old cottages. Each ranch style duplex unit is provided with a "call button" to use in case of medical emergency. Responses are prompt because of the close proximity of the nursing facility.

Residents bring their own furniture when moving into Otterbein. However, no furniture which cannot be adequately stored and suitably arranged within the space available to the residents may be brought.

Health care housing. In addition to the independent living units, the health care unit contains 356 beds defined as either personal care, intermediate care, or skilled nursing care.[3] Albright, Newcomer, and Asbury Halls, built in 1975, provide two levels of intermediate care for over 195 residents (208 if all semi-private). The three 1-story buildings are interconnected. Albright and Asbury Halls are designed for personal care and have a total capacity for 158 residents. Newcomer Hall, with a capacity for 66 residents, provides intermediate nursing care. The second and third floors of the campus center building house the skilled nursing area of 132 beds. Of these nursing beds, two personal care beds and four skilled

---

[3]See "Medical Care" section for definitions of the types of services offered in the health care unit.

nursing beds are left open for immediate use by residents presently living in independent housing. All health care beds are certified for Medicaid while only 132 skilled nursing beds are certified for Medicare.

Costs to residents. Resident are provided with a choice of two payments plans at Otterbein: the straight monthly plan and the Refundable Life Use Fee plan (RLUF). In the straight monthly plan, the full cost of services, care, and facilities in addition to basic housing is paid by the resident each month as long as his or her financial resources are available. This plan is available in all areas of Otterbein.

The RLUF plan operates for residents who initially occupy newly constructed units. The plan is designed to provide Otterbein with capital needed to construct new facilities. For subsequent occupants, the plan is optional. In the event a resident leaves Otterbein within 10 years after occupancy, he or she receives a pro-rata refund. Similarly, in the event of death within 5 years, a pro-rata refund is returned to the resident's estate.

The RLUF plan benefits both Otterbein and its residents. Otterbein receives funds for capital expenditures without having to borrow money from commercial sources at high interest rates; residents benefit by receiving monthly credit for life (up to 1 percent of the RLUF) and by being able to leave Otterbein and receive a partial refund based on their length of residence.

Rates in 1981 under the RLUF plan range from $12,000 for a duplex studio apartment to $48,100 for a large two-bedroom apartment in the new six plex ranch style complex. For residents who pay this fee, the monthly rent or service charge is reduced by up to 1 percent of the RLUF per month for life. For example, the $380 monthly rent for a studio apartment is reduced by about $120 per month. The actual reduction depends on the amount paid and the resident's age at the time of entry.

The cost of independent housing at Otterbein varies according to four factors: 1) the type of unit; 2) the presence or absence of a garage; 3) the number of people living in the unit; and 4) the type of payment plan chosen by the resident.

Whatever combination of housing type, payment plan, etc. the residents choose, the monthly rate for independent housing includes: 1) main meal of the day ($50 per person deducted if not desired); 2) all utilities except telephone; 3) apartment upkeep and repair; 4) program activities; 5) transportation for shopping; 6) insurance of household contents; 7) general upkeep of buildings, grounds, drives; 8) priority use of health care facilities; and 9) $750 worth of health services per year. It should also be noted that it is Otterbein's policy to help the largest possible number of persons who are unable to pay the full cost of services. No one has ever been evicted from Otterbein because he or she lacked funds. The benevolent program is primarily supported by contributions from churches and individuals. Charitable assistance totals over $300,000 per year and serves over 200 residents.

The ranch style duplex apartments are the least expensive of the independent housing units offered at Otterbein. Under the straight monthly plan, a studio apartment for one person with no garage costs $380 per month (1981 rate). A large two-bedroom apartment with a garage for two people costs $814 per month. The costs for these same units under the RLUF plan are either $12,000 (life use fee) plus $260 per month or $27,700 (life use fee) plus about $537 per month.

The independent housing in the two congregate buildings is more costly than the ranch style duplex apartments due to somewhat higher operative costs. Under the straight monthly plan, a standard studio apartment for one person (no garages are available) costs $485 per month (1981 rate). A two-bedroom apartment for two people costs $950 per month. The refundable life use fee rates for these same two apartments range from $14,400 (life use fee) plus $341 per month to $27,500 (life use fee) plus $682 per month.

The projected increase in the costs of the new apartments now under construction reflects sizable increases in construction costs. The initial residents of these units will be required to utilize the refundable life use fee plan. Although Otterbein has been able to keep the monthly rates roughly the same as those of comparable duplexes, the life use fee will be considerably greater ($23,100 versus $12,000 for a studio and $48,100 versus $25,500 for a large two-bedroom).

The costs involved in living in the health care unit depend upon the level of health care required and the payment plan selected by the resident. Skilled nursing care costs about $1,550 per month (semi-private) under the straight monthly rate plan. The cost of intermediate care under the monthly rate plan is about $1,300 per month. Under the RLUF plan, the cost is $11,000 (life use fee) plus about $1,200 per month. Personal care units vary in size and thus in price as well. The least expensive personal care unit is a semi-private room for one person which costs somewhat less than $900 per month under the monthly plan and $11,000 life use fee plus about $775 per month under the RLUF plan. The most expensive personal care unit is a two-room suite for a married couple which costs about $2,300 per couple per month under the monthly plan and $44,000 (life use fee) per couple plus about $2,000 per month under the RLUF plan.

Demand. The Admissions Office compiles and updates a waiting list of all persons who are interested in living at Otterbein. Applicants advance on the list according to a system which gives consideration to the date of the application and need.

As noted earlier, there were 1,800 names on the waiting list during spring, 1981. Approximately 300 names are added to the list each year while roughly 85 persons are accepted for admission per year. Of the 1,800 people waiting for admission, about two-thirds have applied for independent housing. The popularity of independent housing has grown over the past 10 years and, according to the administrators, is attributed to two factors. First, the addition of independent housing has enabled prospective residents to see for themselves that communal living arrangements can co-exist with medical facilities. Second, more people have decided to seek a secure environment prior to their actual need for nursing care.

Over the last 11 years, nearly 1,000 people have been admitted to Otterbein; about one-third to independent housing and two-thirds to health care units. This one-to-two ratio has resulted from the high turnover in the health care unit. The life expectancy of residents moving into the skilled nursing unit is 2 years as compared to 6 years for those in personal care and 10 years for residents in the independent housing units. On the average, there have been 62 deaths annually at Otterbein since 1977.

In light of the different turnover rates and the demand for the various levels of care offered at Otterbein, the waiting period for admittance varies. There is a 6 to 12 month wait for the nursing unit, a 1 year wait for the personal care unit, and a 5 to 8 year wait for independent living units.

Facilities and Services (F/S)

The facilities and services provided at Otterbein reflect a philosophy of self-help and mutual assistance. Otterbein offers a flexible program of services that is capable of responding to the changing interests of its residents. Residents are encouraged to participate in activities and also to assist others in doing so. The success of this mutual help effort is evidenced by the 100,000 hours of volunteered time donated by the residents in 1980.

F/S provided by Otterbein. Otterbein has many facilities that make it possible for residents to conduct their lives without having to ever leave the campus. For example, it has a post office, bank, library, church, general store, clothing store, furniture store, and a soda shop. According to staff, the convenience and opportunity to participate in the operation of the various facilities makes these facilities popular with the residents.

The library contains approximately 5,000 books as well as a large collection of current magazines. It is operated entirely by resident volunteers. The Lebanon Public Library supports the library by loaning it books and by providing a bookmobile once a month.

The Otterbein Home Church, a duly organized United Methodist Church, is on the campus but is independent of it. Approximately 60 percent of the residents and Home employees are members. Weekly attendance numbers around 300 persons.

The clothing store offers residents used clothing for both men and women. The clothing comes from many resources including church groups and individuals. Originally the clothing store gave away pieces of clothing to the residents. This practice was stopped, however, because residents were reluctant to accept clothing if it were given to them. As a result, a minimal charge was asked for clothing; the store is now very popular. It is now thought of as a bargain store and residents boast of the bargains they were able to find. Surplus is put on sale once or twice each year, and may be purchased by employees. The money from these sales is used to purchase other necessities for the Home.

The furniture store enables new residents to sell furniture and household items they cannot use in their apartments or rooms. The store is popular with the residents, employees, and persons living in the surrounding community because of the reasonably priced, high-quality furniture and antiques which can often be found there. The money from these sales is used to purchase necessities for residents.

Through an agreement made with Armco Steel Company, when land was sold to them for the development of a lake in the early 1970s, Otterbein residents are allowed to use a large nearby private park (Armco Recreational Park). Thus, Otterbein relieved itself of park development and maintenance costs.

Other facilities offered at Otterbein include: dining rooms; lounge areas; gathering areas; an arts and crafts area; a darkroom; two greenhouses; space for woodworking, furniture refinishing and painting; a private pond; a large pavilion; and a beauty and barber shop.

F/S provided by governmental/philanthropic organizations. Approximately 200 persons living in the surrounding area do volunteer work at Otterbein. They assist the residents in various ways, such as giving manicures, feeding them, mending their clothes, and shopping for them. A few volunteers also bring their children with them so as to foster interaction between the young and the old.

While Otterbein provides its own maintenance of streets, utilities, refuse collection, and routine security, units of government (Turtle Creek Township or Warren County) are called upon to provide fire and sheriff protection.

F/S provided by Otterbein for surrounding area. Otterbein's intent has been to provide a range of services to Warren County residents and act as a catalyst for other governmental and philanthropic groups to assist elderly residents who live in private housing. However, if county organizations are unable to operate certain programs, then Otterbein becomes directly involved. Several examples of this policy exist. First, Otterbein's program director was instrumental in establishing the Warren County Council on Aging and has served as its president for many years. Also included in its outreach program are out-patient physical therapy, speech and hearing therapy, and participation in a meals-on-wheels program. These services are all consistent with Otterbein's goal of encouraging people to remain in their own homes for as long as possible.

Otterbein also offers a training and education program for professionals in the field of gerontology. These programs are a Nursing Home Area Training Center and a Gerontology Center. These two programs operated 56 different workshops during the 1980 year, serving 2,150 persons.

A summary of the facilities and services provided by Otterbein is illustrated below in Table 6.3.

Medical Care (MC)

MC provided by Otterbein. Otterbein's philosophy of health care is to provide a range of services so as to accommodate people in various stages of physical and psycho-social need. The goal in the

Table 6.3

PROVIDERS OF FACILITIES AND SERVICES
(NON-MEDICAL)

| Location | Retirement Community (Developer/Sponsor/Residents) | | Governmental/ Philanthropic | Entrepreneurial |
	RC Residents	Non-residents		
Inside RC	library church general store clothing store furniture store soda shop recreation park dining rooms arts and crafts rooms greenhouses	training and education program for gerontologists	post office fire protection police protection	bank beauty and barber shops
Outside RC				

health care unit is to return residents to the most active form of living possible or to help them live within the limitations imposed by chronic conditions until death.

As described in the "Housing" section, Otterbein offers three levels of nursing care: personal care (158 beds), intermediate care (66 beds), and skilled nursing (132 beds).[4] Patients are admitted to the health care area from the surrounding area as well as from the independent living areas of Otterbein.

The skilled nursing program is organized so that a licensed nurse is assigned the total 24-hour responsibility for the care of a resident for as long as that resident resides in the skilled nursing facility. A licensed nurse plans for 16 or 17 residents and gives complete care to four persons while a primary aide assists her in the program. Those on other shifts carry on the plan of care and are known as alternate nurses and aides.

In an effort to allow older people to remain in their own homes as long as possible, outreach programs such as Meals-on-Wheels are available to the surrounding community. Similar services are provided to Otterbein residents as well. For example, residents of the personal care area are encouraged to eat meals in the dining room. However, if a resident is unable to do so, yet a move to intermediate care is not warranted, then meals are served in the small nearby dining hall area. This policy explains why only 7 percent of the residents currently in the nursing care area moved there from independent housing in Otterbein.

A health care insurance policy is available to residents. The policy is for $750 worth of health services per year at a cost of less than $15 per month to the resident.

A summary of the health care services provided by Otterbein is shown in Table 6.4.

Ownership/Management/Governance

Type of ownership. Although Otterbein is related to the West Ohio Conference of the United Methodist Church, the Church is not legally required to support Otterbein's operation. Otterbein is a

---

[4]Skilled nursing care is defined by a full range of 24-hour direct medical, nursing, and other health services. Intermediate care also involves 24-hour service, but with physicians and nurses in a supervisory role. Personal or sheltered care is offered to residents having no serious health problem but who nonetheless have chronic or debilitating conditions requiring assistance with daily activities.

Table 6.4

PROVIDERS OF MEDICAL CARE

Location	Retirement Community (Developer/Sponsor/Residents)		Other Providers (Govt./Philanthropies/Private)
	RC Residents	Non-residents	
Inside RC	personal care beds intermediate care skilled nursing care health care insurance	outreach programs out-patient physical therapy out-patient speech and hearing training	
Outside RC		meals-on-wheels	hospitals ambulances

separate "not-for-profit" corporation. The Church is related to Otterbein in two ways: 1) the Church provides annual contributions to Otterbein; and 2) Otterbein raises funds through the Church's constituency.

Type of management/governance. The Board of Trustees selected by the Conference has the responsibility of hiring an administrator to manage Otterbein. The administrator is responsible for total oversight, including hiring of all other personnel.

Degree of resident involvement. Residents have a voice in the management of Otterbein through a system of counterpart committees. There is now a counterpart committee for each committee of the Board of Trustees. Through these committees, residents may voice complaints or make suggestions for change. Four such committees currently exist: 1) campus property; 2) development; 3) finance and personnel; and 4) resident services. There is also a "Residents' Rights" Committee which enables grievances to be filed under a "Resident's Bill of Rights."

There is also a Resident's Council at Otterbein, but it has no official governing power. The primary function of the Resident's Council is to foster resident activity and participation. There are 14 committees dealing with everything from gardening to the Hobby Lobby Craft Center. Each of these committees is composed of 5 to 10 members; there are as many as 30 to 400 residents participating directly in these activities.

Financing

During the past 10 years, Otterbein has invested nearly 9 million dollars in new operating facilities or major improvements. As an example, a recent year's (1981) operating expenses were approximately $6,000,000. The following sources were used to finance the capital improvements: 1) the refundable life use fee program raised $2,700,000; 2) $1,700,000 was raised in gifts; 3) $600,000 was raised in the form of a Hill-Burton Grant; and 4) bond and note issues covered the $4,000,000 in borrowed funds needed. Operating expenses are covered by the monthly payments of Otterbein residents, Medicaid, Medicare, and benevolent care funds.

Taxes are another expense which Otterbein must incur. Otterbein pays a total of $7,000 to $8,000 yearly in taxes. Property taxes paid by Otterbein are affected by their non-profit status—all land is tax exempt except that which houses employees and leased farm land.

In terms of school taxes, the residents of Otterbein have consistently voted for school bond issues. This indicates a willingness to support the activities and operations of the surrounding community. Discussions with officials at the Warren County Zoning Office and the Warren County Housing Authority suggest that the voting behavior of area residents has not changed over the years.

Marketing and Plans for the Future

Advertising. In light of their waiting list with 1,800 names, Otterbein does not formally advertise. There is, however, an active public relations operation which has the major function of raising funds. Public relations activities include speaking in area churches and publication and distribution of an Otterbein newspaper (The Vista from Otterbein Home). The newspaper is published four times a year and is intended to acquaint readers with the developments and happenings of Otterbein. It is distributed to a mailing list of over 50,000. These public relations activities provide continued support for Otterbein.

Future plans. Otterbein's future plans call for its continued expansion so as to provide for the growing number of people waiting to be admitted. To guide the implementation of this growth, a physical Master Plan has been developed. This plan has been prepared by the Long-Range Planning Committee of the Board of Trustees and provides for the addition of two more campuses adjacent to the present development on land owned by Otterbein. Two new campuses are proposed instead of merely expanding the existing campus so as to maintain the small scale of the Otterbein complex. This decision is in keeping with the philosophy of Otterbein's design. Thus, the Master Plan represents an attempt to grow so as to accommodate the increasing demand while not sacrificing the relatively small, intimate scale of the existing campus. The Home also continually monitors needs in other areas of the Conference and advises on the development of new facilities.

The two new campuses proposed in the Master Plan are similar to the present campus in that the complete range of health care is to be provided. There is a slight difference however. The present campus is 60 percent nursing and 40 percent independent housing. The new campuses are proposed for 40 percent nursing and 60 percent independent housing. This change is the result of the change in the nature of demand as evidenced by the waiting list. The new duplex apartments on the existing campus are viewed as an attraction for prospective residents, many of whom had been hesitant to move into a facility dominated by nursing.

In the Fall of 1980, construction began on the second campus. Occupancy of the first apartments is planned for late 1981 or early 1982. The approximately 150 additional residents will increase Otterbein's total population to about 700 residents.

Plans for the new campuses also reflect Otterbein's desire to be flexible. More congregate apartments without kitchen facilities have been planned since these units can readily be converted into nursing units. Thus, the 33 planned congregate–no cooking apartments could be converted to a 66-bed nursing unit if demand so dictated.

Overview—Impacts of Change

In discussions with the staff and residents, it was learned that the current and planned construction is worrisome to some of the residents. Fears focus on the concern that Otterbein will become too large. Some residents believe they will no longer know and recognize others as they have been able to do in the past. Expansion would diminish the home-like atmosphere and sense of belonging that currently exists. Therefore, Otterbein appears to be nearing another crucial phase in its evolution. Otterbein is faced with the problem of how to accommodate the increasing number of people requesting admission while not sacrificing the small community atmosphere which largely accounts for its current success.

The effects of changes in Otterbein on its residents largely concern the rapid growth of the retirement community over the past decade. Otterbein has more than tripled in size since 1970 and has developed a Master Plan for the development of two new campuses which will triple its size again.

The buildings and site have been designed so as to preserve the small community atmosphere and scale of the 1960s. These efforts have been successful thus far since Otterbein seems to be sociologically as well as physically subdivided into neighborhood units.

Another change which has occurred in Otterbein over the past 10 years concerns the increase in the amount of independent living units available. The ratio of health care units to independent units has changed from 6-to-1 in 1970 to 1.5-to-1 in 1980. Such change might be expected to create a shift in the average age of the residents of Otterbein. On the contrary, Otterbein has remained a retirement community for the older elderly (over 75) who seem to be seeking the security offered by health care facilities. This implies that the mere provision of independent housing units does not necessarily attract the young, healthy older person. Instead, it appears to be a combination of housing type, recreational facilities, and services, and the emphasis of health care relative to independent living.

Otterbein seems to have had a limited impact on its surroundings. This is attributable to the geographic isolation of Otterbein and the large amount of undeveloped land which separates it from the outside community. The County Planner and officials at the County Housing Authority indicated that Otterbein had no impact on the surrounding area. However, according to an administrator, local merchants in the area immediately surrounding Otterbein realize a substantial economic benefit from the patronage of residents and over 330 full- or part-time employees who spend much of the $3.2 million payroll in the local area.

Summary

Otterbein has evolved through various phases of development since its inception. It began in 1913 as a County Poor House for both children and older people and did not become a continuing care retirement community until the mid-1960s. The concept of the refundable life use fee payment plan was also introduced in the 1960s. Prior to that time, older residents were required to surrender their financial assets upon admission. Over the past 20 years, Otterbein has grown in size and now offers housing for independent living as well as three levels of nursing care. The retirement center is currently entering yet another phase with the development of one and possibly two new adjoining campuses. With this expansion, the size of Otterbein's population could double or triple. The expected growth could have negative and positive effects on Warren County and nearby Lebanon, Ohio. The County could lose property revenue as a result of Otterbein's growth and removal of land from the tax rolls. At the same time, the increase in population could benefit commerce in Lebanon and elsewhere in the County. If Otterbein were to double or triple in size, a major challenge will be the preservation of the small community atmosphere it has enjoyed over the years.

Chapter 7

Summary and Conclusions

In this final chapter an overview is presented of the detailed information contained in the preceding case studies. For the sake of clarity, we have organized this rather unwieldy collection of information into two sections. First, we synthesize the present state of retirement communities with respect to our typology. Second, we identify five principle ways in which retirement communities have changed or evolved. These two sections serve to develop and explain the characteristics and experiences of retirement communities.

The Present State of Retirement Communities

As we indicated earlier, most retirement communities that exist in the United States today can be categorized according to one of five types: new towns, villages, subdivisions, residences, and continuing care retirement centers. The current status of retirement communities is discussed by addressing each of these community types.

New Towns

Retirement new towns are designed for retirees interested in both a leisurely and active life-style within a self-contained community setting. These privately built developments, aimed at both the preretirement and retirement market, are most commonly found in Sunbelt and western states so as to take advantage of a climate conducive to year-round outdoor activity.

As noted earlier, the new town is the largest of the retirement communities. They have a population of at least 5,000 residents, although many are considerably larger. For example, the 1981 populations of two well-publicized retirement new towns, Arizona's Sun City and California's Leisure World, were 47,500 and 22,000, respectively. Such communities occupy large tracts of several thousand acres.

Various housing options are available to prospective new town residents. Single-family homes, two and four plex housing, and townhouses abound. High-rise buildings, designed for residents seeking security and continuing health care, may also be found in new towns. In addition to fee simple ownership such as available in Sun City and Sun City Center, condominium and cooperative living arrangements are available. In fact, all housing within California's Leisure World is sold as cooperatives and condominiums.

Since new towns are designed to be virtually self-contained, numerous support services and facilities are included as part of the community. In fact, when compared to other types of retirement communities, new towns offer the most extensive network of recreational, commercial, financial, and medical services. Opportunities for both active and passive recreational pursuits are abundant. For example, Sun City, Arizona contains 11 golf courses, 8 lawn bowling greens, 72 shuffleboard courts, 4 miniature golf courses, 7 swimming pools, and 17 tennis courts. In addition, there are 5 auditoriums, while studios and game rooms are available for hobbies, crafts, or other activities, such as billiards, table tennis, and cards.

Facilities within the community for shopping, banking, and dining out are also plentiful, making it convenient for residents to conduct personal affairs. Sun City, for instance, contains six shopping centers with a total of over 350 shops and businesses, and 16 restaurants, gas stations, and local newspapers. Sun City Center has one shopping center while Leisure World, California contains small shopping centers with numerous shops and commercial establishments. Financial institutions are commonly found in new towns as well. In Sun City, there are 16 branch banks and 25 savings and loan associations.

A range of health care and medical facilities are also available in new towns. Sun City, Arizona and Leisure World, California even contain hospitals. If hospitals are not available within the new town, they are likely to be located nearby. Medical clinics housing doctors' offices and laboratories are often located within new towns as well. Some new towns may even contain nursing homes or continuing care retirement centers. For example, there are two continuing care centers in Sun City, Arizona and two more are adjacent to the retirement community.

Two distinct philosophies of security are reflected in the physical design of new towns. One is represented by the closed, self-contained community and is characterized by perimeter walls and security gates restricting access to the development. This philosophy is reflected in the layout of Leisure World, California. The other philosophy may be characterized as an open community, undifferentiated from its surroundings and having unrestrictive access. Sun City, Arizona is reflective of this philosophy.

New town retirees tend to be young and active retirement aged people seeking involvement in various forms of active recreational and leisure pursuits. The only restrictions placed on residency in most new towns is a minimum age; residents typically must be over 50 years old.

The average age of residents is generally less than 75 years. However, in some new towns, residents are much younger. For example, the typical resident in Sun City Center is 64 years old while in Leisure World, California, the average age of residents is 73 years old. Households, for the most part, consist of couples having middle and upper middle-income backgrounds. Although fewer than one-third of the residents work either full- or part-time, many are involved in voluntary organizations and activities within the retirement community.

New towns attract people from all parts of the country. However, the specific market area for any particular town will vary depending on its location. Sun City and Sun City Center, Florida, for example, attract a national market with the midwest states being the largest supplier of residents. Others, such as the Leisure Worlds, attract most of their residents from the local region.

The different market areas and housing tenure arrangements also reflect the seasonality of new town residents. In Sun City and Sun City Center, about one-third of the residents move away during the summer months. However, two-thirds of the residents in the condominium development within Sun City Center (King's Point) are seasonal. In contrast, virtually all of the residents in California's Leisure World are year-rounders.

New towns are typically the creation of large development corporations owning or holding options on large parcels of land. Generally, they are built in stages. The timing of construction within each stage is a function of home sales, which vary with marketing efforts, interest rates, and the general state of the economy. Often, recreational lands and facilities, roads, and other services are created prior to housing. This occurred in the three new towns we visited.

Major trends in new towns. Since retirement new towns are com-

monly developed in stages, the character of each stage is largely a
reflection of changes in the market and in the developer's philosophy. One change that has occurred in new town development over
the past decade has been the increased size of new home construction. For the most part, new town developers have built larger and
more expensive homes as the community entered its later stages. In
response to double digit inflation and high interest rates, which in-
hibit the purchase of homes by the middle-income elderly,
developers have built houses appealing to people with higher incomes. In Sun City, for example, the original plan aimed at attracting middle-income retirees. Housing of about 1,000 square feet cost
$11,000 in 1960; by 1980, the average cost of a new 2,000 square
feet house was nearly $100,000. Under these circumstances, resi-
dents attracted to the community over the period of development
have been increasingly affluent.

In addition to rising housing costs and the increased size of new
dwellings, new towns are characterized by aging segments of their
populations and, concurrently, changes in their service requirements. For the most part, new towns have been able to avoid an increasing average age of their residents. However, portions of the established populations age along with the retirement community
itself. As a result, services catering to the medical needs of the population have been introduced in recent years. Herein lies an interesting paradox in the evolution of retirement new towns. The developers feel that introducing nursing and medical facilities early in
the development process adversely affects the image of an active retirement community, and therefore discourages younger and more
affluent retirees from moving in. On the other hand, established
residents argue that the developer is not just building houses and
recreation centers, but is actually creating a community that would
be incomplete without facilities for health care required by residents
as they grow older. Although there appears to be no "formula" by
which to respond to this dilemma, it is nonetheless a problem that
must be addressed in the development of new towns for retirees.

Retirement Village

These retirement communities are intended to house a retirement
and pre-retirement population in a secure setting offering a wide
assortment of leisure and recreational activities. Unlike new towns,

retirement villages are not planned to be self-contained communities. Rather, they are located in urbanizing areas containing a full range of services from which the retirement community and its residents can draw. Although commonly found in Sunbelt states, villages have also been built in northern states.

Retirement villages are smaller than new towns—generally ranging in size from 1,000 to 5,000 people. Housing type, quantity, and density can vary greatly, both within and between communities. Options include single-family detached homes, 2-8 plexes, low-rise and high-rise apartment buildings, and mobile homes. Leisure World, Maryland, Leisure World, California, and Leisure Village West in New Jersey each provide a combination of housing types. In contrast, Country Village Apartments and Hawthorne offer only one type of housing—low-rise apartment buildings and mobile homes, respectively. Typically, mobile homes are not mixed with conventionally built housing and some developers prefer greater uniformity of housing type within one community to reduce costs. Given the variation in housing and density of development, it is not uncommon for retirement villages to occupy as little as 100 acres of land, such as Country Village Apartments, or as much as 1,200 acres.

There is also variability in the forms of housing tenure in retirement villages. In addition to traditional fee-simple ownership, cooperative and condominium arrangements (Leisure World, Maryland, Leisure Village, and Leisure Village West), rentals (Country Village Apartments), and mobile home ownership combined with lot rental (Hawthorne) are available in retirement villages. Regardless of tenure arrangement, residents typically pay a monthly fee to cover the operating costs of selected community services.

As mentioned earlier, recreational and communal facilities and programs are prevalent in retirement villages. Indoor facilities typically include a clubhouse with rooms for meetings, performances, crafts, games, and an assortment of classes. Outside facilities include swimming pools, golf course(s), shuffleboard courts, and tennis courts. In short, the recreation/leisure facilities of a village often rival those found in new towns.

Because retirement villages are not planned to be self-contained communities, the extent to which they provide shopping facilities either on-site or on the perimeter of the village varies. Some villages, such as Leisure World, Maryland, contain a few private businesses. Others have commercial establishments adjoining their perimeter. Still others, such as Hawthorne, contain no commercial facilities and are fairly distant from the nearest shopping.

Similarly, the provision of health care facilities and services varies among retirement villages. Most villages offer only emergency medical service. However, Leisure World, Maryland contains a medical clinic with physicians, dentists, laboratory facilities, a pharmacy, and an emergency service and home visiting service. In contrast, Country Village Apartments provides only limited health care (a monthly screening clinic).

As in the case of new towns, retirement villages differ from one another in the extent to which security is available. Many are surrounded by walls with guarded entrances to limit access to residents and authorized visitors. In all retirement villages we visited, this type of extensive security was present.

Like new towns, retirement villages tend to attract young, active, and gregarious residents. Residence in many is limited to people in their early 50s, although some, such as Country Village Apartments, are age-integrated communities. For the most part, the population in retirement villages consists of retired couples in their late 60s, who are college educated and financially comfortable. Not all retirement villages, however, house an affluent and well educated population. In Country Village Apartments, for example, social security is the major source of income for half of the residents, and many have no more than a high school education.

Major trends in retirement villages. The overall pattern of aging among retirement village residents has been similar to that occurring in new towns. Although the average age of residents has remained fairly constant over the years, a subset of residents has aged. The manner in which the changing service needs of aging village residents are dealt with is slightly different than in new towns. Unlike new towns which are planned as self-contained communities, retirement villages are most likely to utilize services from the surrounding area. Consequently, as the service requirements of village populations have changed, villages have responded differently. For example, some, such as Hawthorne, have adopted firm policies that no nursing care will be introduced in the village, forcing residents to move who no longer can live independently. On the other hand, other developers have provided supportive housing within the village setting so as to accommodate the changing needs of the aging residents. The more supportive housing often is in the form of high-rise apartment buildings offering meal and maid service. In Leisure

World, Maryland, the Rossmoor Corporation is contemplating the building of a continuing care facility.

Another trend in the evolution of retirement villages is their attraction of more affluent residents as the community has matured. This is mainly due to two factors. First, as the costs of providing services increases, monthly fees must be raised, services must be eliminated, or a change to fee-for-service must be instituted on services previously included in the monthly charge. As a result, it has become increasingly expensive to live in a retirement village. Higher housing costs have, in turn, discouraged many people from moving to retirement villages while attracting affluent retirees. A second factor leading to the increasing affluence of new residents concerns people's buying habits. According to one village developer, people with higher incomes tend to wait before purchasing homes in new developments until the developments are shown to be successful. The developer thus views increasing affluence among new residents as a typical and expected pattern.

There has also been a tendency for retirement villages offering cooperative and/or condominium ownership to experience difficulties during the transition of control from the developer to residents. Developers generally agree to transfer control of a development to the residents upon completion of a specified amount of the village and/or by a specified date. However, many of these agreements were made before the rapid climb in interest rates which often either slowed or curtailed development altogether. This slowdown of development has often created tension between the developer and residents. Residents may seek to force the developer to complete the village as planned or even to alter the original plan so as to better fit their demands. The developer, on the other hand, is often reluctant to relinquish control before the development is substantially completed for fear that resident control would result in a less profitable development.

Subdivisions

Retirement subdivisions are privately built residential environments, planned for a predominantly independent elderly population. In contrast to new towns and retirement villages, they contain a limited number of services and facilities for resident use. Consequently, they are planned as part of the fabric of the surrounding environment which is usually rich in services and amenities. The larger community then becomes the major attraction for prospective residents who seek a living arrangement unencumbered by a costly infra-structure, which contains for the most part older people. Retirement subdivisions, therefore, tend to be located in the urban areas of Florida and other Sunbelt states so as to take advantage of the attractive climate. Their size varies, although most house no more than 500 persons.

Community services and facilities in subdivisions are usually limited to a small meeting room or recreation center. Orange Gardens, for example, contains only a meeting room and a small library in a community house. However, some subdivisions contain more extensive recreational and leisure facilities. For example, Trailer Estates has an auditorium, meeting and game rooms, 32 shuffleboard courts, a marina, a private beach on Sarosata Bay, a laundromat, and their own volunteer fire department. Commercial, medical, or nursing facilities/services are typically not available within retirement subdivisions but usually are in abundance throughout the surrounding environment. Compared to the other classes of retirement communities, subdivisions represent the least supportive form of retirement living from a facility perspective.

Subdivisions tend to be characterized by either of two housing types: conventionally built single-family homes or mobile homes. In subdivisions containing conventionally built homes, such as Orange Gardens, residents are likely to own their dwellings, whereas tenure arrangements vary in mobile home developments. In some places, the home and lot are both owned (Trailer Estates), whereas in other places, the mobile home is purchased by the resident who rents the lot from the developer (Bradenton Trailer Park and Riviera Mobile Home Park). Ownership of home and lot is a relatively new option for residents of mobile home retirement subdivisions. Trailer Estates, a mobile home park near Bradenton, Florida, was the first development to offer this form of ownership in 1955.

Although many subdivisions impose limitations on the age of prospective residents, many do not or will only allow adults 18 years of age or older. For example, residents of Riviera Mobile Home Park must be at least 50 years of age, while Bradenton Trailer Park only requires residents to be adults (18 years old). Still others, such as Trailer Estates, have sections of the development set aside for young couples, while some, such as Orange Gardens, permit families with school age children. Most retirement subdivisions, however, house a predominantly older population; the majority of their residents are retired and were attracted to the community by its relatively homogeneous environment and modest cost of living. Even Orange Gardens, which has not had an age limitation for residency since it opened in 1954, has maintained a predominantly over-50 population.

Older residents in retirement subdivisions are similar in many respects to residents of new towns and retirement villages. Households generally consist of married couples in their early 70s, both of whom are in good health. Many residents are employed either full- or part-time, and, unlike those in new towns and villages, several remain active in the host community. This pattern of involvement is consistent with the nature of subdivisions: to be an integral part of the surrounding environment.

In general, the populations of subdivisions tend to be less affluent than those in new towns or retirement villages. Since retirement subdivisions contain fewer services and many are mobile home parks, they are more affordable than the other types of large-scale retirement communities. Retirement subdivisions are sometimes referred to as the "bargain" retirement communities of the South.

Subdivisions are generally developed by for-profit developers. One exception to this rule is the Bradenton Trailer Park of Bradenton, Florida, which is owned and operated by the local Kiwanis Club. However, it is the only trailer park owned by a service organization in the country.

Retirement subdivisions are viewed as attractive business ventures for small developers. Whereas new towns and villages require large initial capital investments so as to construct recreation and service facilities, subdivisions can be developed with a relatively small intial capital investment because they contain few such facilities.

Major trends in subdivisions. Since subdivisions provide few services and facilities, the major trends that have occurred in their evolution and maturation concern the residents. The average age of residents seems to have remained stable if not decreased. It seems that residents tend to move to more medically supportive environments when their health begins to deteriorate, thus preventing the average age from drastically increasing. This phenomenon seems to be more characteristic of mobile home subdivisions than conventionally built subdivisions. This is probably due to accessibility problems of most mobile homes, making them difficult to negotiate in failing health.

Since many subdivisions do not restrict residency to those over 50 years of age, there is also a possibility that the average age of residents may be reduced as more younger people move in. However, this does not seem to be a common trend. It seems that the services and facilities offered by a retirement subdivision, combined with specialized advertising directed at a retirement age clientele, generally attract people over 50 years of age.

Retirement Residences

These small retirement communities are supportive environments designed to accommodate a relatively independent life-style at a moderate cost to older retired persons. They are likely to be built under the sponsorship of non-profit groups, such as churches, unions, or benevolent organizations. Residences are typically located in urban areas near public transportation, shopping, and medical services, and are found in all parts of the United States.

To a large extent, residences are small communities of older people, often housed in a single high-rise building. Many have been designed as apartment hotels and, over time, have attained retirement community stature by virtue of change in ownership. For example, Williams Memorial Residence is housed in the former Hotel Marcy, a residential hotel in New York City. Residences, on the average, contain fewer than 500 dwelling units, most of which are apartments rented on a month-to-month basis. Charges to residents cover meals and sometimes services such as laundry and transportation. Besides apartments, retirement residences contain communal rooms and dining facilities, where residents may be required to eat at least one meal per day. Other meals are taken in apartments having small kitchenettes.

Residences are similar to subdivisions in that they generally lack outdoor recreational facilities such as golf courses, tennis courts, and swimming pools. At the same time, their social programs and the indoor facilities to accommodate them may be similar to, although less extensive, than those found in retirement villages, or even new towns. These facilities might include lounges, craft areas and/or game rooms, and multi-purpose rooms. Planned programs, organized by resident staff, typically include classes, parties, lectures, and excursions to places in the surrounding area.

Another characteristic common to both retirement residences and subdivisions is their lack of health care facilities and services. Apartments in retirement residences, however, are often equipped with emergency call buttons, while staff is sometimes trained in emergency medical techniques.

People living in residences tend to be older than those found in new towns, villages, and subdivisions. The typical resident is a single woman, around 75 years old, white, and living on a modest income. She, like her neighbors, is generally in good health and independent. She leaves the residence when she wishes and rarely seeks assistance from the staff. She was attracted to the residence by its relatively modest cost, its security, its services, and potential for finding companionship.

For the most part, residents have lived in a private home or apartment elsewhere in the host community or region prior to their moving to the retirement residence. Nearly all residents of Williams Memorial Residence and Baptist Gardens had previously lived in the New York City area and Long Beach, California area, respectively. In many cases, residents continue to maintain contact with the outside world by participating in church activities, or by doing volunteer work in nearby schools and hospitals. Most, however, remain close to their new community where programs such as coffee hours, classes, and other get-togethers are plentiful. Besides their participating in activities organized by the retirement community, residents sometimes plan and carry out their own group activities without the assistance of the resident staff.

Staff size in retirement residences is usually small. They are likely to be hired by a Board of Directors which is a creation of the sponsor. In planning the building retirement residences, many non-profit sponsors are assisted by federal programs which provide direct loans at lower rates than would otherwise be available. Baptist Gardens was built with the assistance of Section 236 federal monies. Under this program, a non-profit sponsor as well as a limited dividend developer could build rental housing with an interest subsidy dependent on the incomes of tenants accepted into the housing. Thus, housing costs are maintained at relatively low levels, thereby attracting households with limited financial resources. In contrast, it is necessary for the Salvation Army-sponsored Williams Memorial Residence to charge residents for the full cost of housing and services, since it operates without a government subsidy or aid from the Salvation Army.

Major trends in retirement residences. Retirement residences typically provide a constant, stable living environment for their older tenants. Many, built during the 1950s and 1960s, are characterized by an aging population having greater health care and social service needs. In efforts to preserve the original character of the community and its residents, while at the same time minimizing the rate of increase in operating costs, some residences have altered policies so as to attract young retirees. Williams Memorial Residence, for example, lowered the minimum age for admission from 65 to 55. Others, such as Baptist Gardens, have not adapted to the changing requirements of their tenants. By not doing so, the increasingly dependent elderly have been forced to seek alternative living arrangements. For many, the move has been a disruptive force in their lives. In other retirement residences, however, policies of accommodating to the changing requirements of tenants have been established. Williams Memorial Residence modified policies so as to allow residents to hire their own nursing aides so they may remain in the residence even after they require the assistance of limited nursing care. It is also possible for retirement residences to satisfy the changing needs of residents through environmental modification and introduction of health care and other supportive services.

Continuing Care Retirement Centers

Unlike retirement residences, these retirement communities provide a medically supportive environment, based on a concept of continuing health care. Health care is offered to older persons from their early, independent retirement years to a period when they are totally dependent. These communities enable an older person to live a completely independent life-style while being assured that health care and social support are available at a later stage in life.

Continuing care centers generally operate under non-profit sponsorship. They tend to be located in urban areas, although some are situated in rural settings. As in the case of retirement residences, these communities are found in all parts of the United States. Compared to new towns and villages, continuing care retirement centers are small. They seldom exceed 1,000 residents, with most containing fewer than 500 residents.

Residents of continuing care retirement centers are housed in either a complex of buildings or sometimes in a single building. The building complex typically contains a mix of residential structures and dining facilities, meeting rooms, and medical facilities. Residential structures can range from congregate apartment buildings to independent cottages and townhouses. Otterbein Home, Presbyterian Home, and Sunny Shores Villas each consist of a complex of buildings. When a continuing care retirement center consists of a single structure, all medical facilities, housing units, and support services are housed under one roof. Friendship Village is such a retirement community. It is housed in a 3-story building which is divided into six pavilions, or interconnected clusters of residential units. Residents are able to walk anywhere in the retirement community without having to go out-of-doors. There are also numerous informal gathering places in the building with views to the outside and ample opportunities for residents to walk or congregate out-of-doors.

The services in continuing care requirement centers are predominantly nursing and/or medical in nature. They are designed to accommodate people needing various levels of physical and social support. Many retirement centers offer three levels of nursing care: skilled, intermediate, and personal care.[1] In addition, these retirement communities may contain an infirmary for temporary nursing care. To staff these facilities, an assortment of health care professionals is needed, including nurses, physical therapists, social workers, and physicans. Due to the wide assortment of supportive services provided in continuing care retirement centers, they have the highest resident-to-staff ratio of any of the five retirement community types. In the centers we visited, ratios ranged from 15:1 to 3:1.

In addition to medical and social services, continuing care retirement centers offer numerous opportunities for social and recreational pursuits. Many have facilities and programs for arts and crafts, games, classes, billiards, and choral groups. As in the case of the retirement residences, they rarely have facilities for active outdoor sports such as golfing, tennis, and swimming. Most continuing care communities contain a congregate dining area, snack bars, a library, a chapel, a beauty/barber shop serviced at specified times throughout the week, lounges for informal gathering, and sometimes a gift shop and small convenience grocery.

Continuing care retirement centers have more restrictive admissions requirements than other types of retirement communities. In addition to a minimum age, usually over 50, applicants must meet specified health and financial standards. In most cases, prospective residents must demonstrate at entry an ability to live independently

---

[1]Skilled nursing care is defined by a full range of 24-hour direct medical, nursing, and other health services. Intermediate care also involves 24-hour service, but with physicians and nurses in a supervisory role. Personal or sheltered care is offered to residents having no serious health problem but who nonetheless have chronic or debilitating conditions requiring assistance with daily activities.

for a certain period of time, say 3 to 5 years, and to afford the endowment and the monthly fees for several years.

Residents on the average are older than those found in other types of retirement communities. The typical resident of a retirement center is likely to be an elderly woman in her late 70s or early 80s and widowed. She comes from either a middle or upper-middle class background. Couples occupy a small proportion of the dwellings, and in rare cases, the husband continues to work, usually on a part-time basis. Few residents leave the community for prolonged periods.

The motives of residents who move to a continuing care center differ from the motives of people attracted to new towns, villages, and subdivisions. Continuing care residents are motivated by the security, both medical and financial, offered by this living arrangement. In contrast, retirees choosing new towns, villages, or retirement subdivisions are attracted by the opportunities for maintaining or beginning an active life of leisure. Most continuing care residents had made the decision not to move away from home during their younger retirement years, but later decided to move into a more secure environment as they grew older. However, even then they tend to remain close to home. Thus, most residents of continuing care communities formerly lived in the local area. In fact, continuing care centers and residences have the smallest market area of the five classes of retirement communities.

Most continuing care retirement centers require residents to enter into some form of life-care contract. By entering into this contract, they are assigned an independent living unit and have access to nursing care whenever needed. The life care contract usually involves the payment of an initial endowment or founder's fee plus a monthly fee. The endowment fee is usually either non-refundable, or only partially refundable if the resident decides to leave or dies within a limited period. The amount of endowment or founder's fees varies considerably between and within communities, depending on its location and the size and type of living unit. A few years ago, it was not uncommon to find endowment fees ranging from $10,000 to $75,000 while monthly maintenance fees varied from $200 to $2,000. In many continuing care centers built and operated under the sponsorship of benevolent groups, a small portion of the residents receive public assistance.

The life-care concept is also based on the notion of pre-paid health care. In addition to the endowment fee which may be used for this purpose, residents who live independently generally pay higher monthly fees than the cost of services they receive. By doing so, they are able to pay less than the acutal cost of services they receive when they move into the health care unit of the community. This pre-payment policy serves to stabilize monthly payments for residents. It also means that if a resident does not live independently long enough to sufficiently pre-pay for health care to be recieved later, the retirement community must subsidize the resident. Thus, continuing care retirement centers offering life-care contacts have a vested interest in admitting residents who will be able to live independently for a number of years before needing nursing care.

There are also many continuing care retirement centers that do not offer life-care contracts. These communities would be classified as retirement residences except that they provide health care, either long- or short-term. For example, Trinity Lakes in Sun City, Florida and The Shores in Bradenton, Florida are sheltered care facilities which each include a health and therapy center. Most often, the health care facilities and services provided in these communities are not as extensive as in those offering life-care contracts. Thus, residents are guaranteed health care for only as long as the facility is capable of caring for the resident. Few residents are forced to leave for health reasons. In addition, health care services are provided on a fee-for-service basis. These communities also generally require residents to pay a membership fee which is similar to the endowment fees required by life-care communities.

Major trends in continuing care retirement centers. Two related trends in the evolution of continuing care retirement centers have been identified. First, the average age of residents has tended to increase as the existing residents grow older and the average age of new applicants rises. Many retirement centers have difficulty attracting younger independent residents, in part because older people are unlikely to consider a move to a continuing care community until they recognize the possibility of failing health.

Second, in the continuing care centers with life-care contracts, the nature and content of these contracts have changed over time. As the populations of these communities age, the period of time residents are able to live independently decreases. As a result, many do not sufficiently "pre-pay" for their future health care expenses. This phenomenon, coupled with rapidly rising medical costs, has prompted many continuing care retirement centers to alter their life-care contracts, which placed ceilings on the annual increase in monthly fees. In response to this problem, many retirement centers have written new contracts to substantially increase the amount of possible increases or eliminate limitations altogether. In this way, the communities are able to pass on the increasing health care costs to the residents. However, retirement centers still honor older contracts, causing cash-flow problems for many of them.

In sum, continuing care retirement centers have experienced an aging of their populations and rising medical costs. For those offering life-care contracts, the response has been changing contractual arrangements. Most life-care communities seem to be adjusting successfully despite the fact that they must subsidize residents with older contracts having low ceilings on permissible cost increases. For continuing care retirement centers not offering life-care contracts, this has not been as serious a problem, since health care services are provided on a fee-for-service basis.

Changing Properties of Retirement Communities

Our study of these retirement communities, together with the review of the literature, clearly indicate that although retirement communities are dynamic organizations which change over time, the nature and timing of the changes vary between and within each class. As part of our work, we have identified five principle ways in which retirement communities, taken as a whole, have changed since their inception. We note that a number of these changing characteristics or properties are interrelated and may not be applicable to every retirement community in existence. Even in our study of a small sample of communities, we have found anomalies. Nonetheless, we consider these five properties to be important and generally characteristic of most retirement communities that exist in the United States today. In the discussion which follows, we point out some of the specific changes experienced within different classes of retirement communities and the manner in which our sample communities and their residents have responded to these changes. In some instances, one changing property may be considered a response to one or more of the other changing properties. For example, in some classes of communities, shifts in patterns of retirement community governance may be considered a response to both rising costs and retirement community growth and expansion. The five changing properties are:

1. Segments of the resident population of retirement communities age.
2. Retirement communities grow in size and scope.
3. Changes occur in the physical, political, and socioeconomic character of the surroundings within which retirement communities are located.
4. Retirement communities experience rising costs resulting from inflation which impact on their operations and on their residents.
5. Retirement communities experience changes in governance and management.

Segments of the population age. In a number of our case studies, we identified members of the population who had lived in the retirement community since its inception. In some communities, for example, residents who moved in when they were in their 50s are now in their 70s; in other communities, residents who were 70 are now in their 80s or even older. In many instances, this aging process was accompanied by a trend toward an older population. Whereas the average age in the community was 60 at one time, it may now be 75. In other cases, however, the average age of the community has remained constant over time or has even declined. In part, the declining average age is the result of younger people having entered the community in recent years. Yet, there are many long-term residents of such communities who have aged.

Among the aging population, most are widows, with few being employed. For many, their involvement in community activities declines as they grow older and experience declining health. Generally, these aging residents are less mobile than they had once been within the community setting. At the same time, their need for various supportive services has changed, particularly with respect to housing, health care, transportation, and social/recreational activity.

Our study has shown that retirement new towns are most adaptive to these changing needs. With respect to health care, new facilities such as hospitals and programs such as homemaker services have been introduced, often at the instigation of the residents (Sun City, Leisure World, California). In some cases, the private sector has responded to these changing needs either within or adjacent to the new towns. Private developers and non-profit groups have built retirement residences (Leisure World, California) and continuing care centers (Sun City, Sun City Center), designed to accommodate the need for more sheltered living arrangements, smaller independent housing units, health care and, in general, a more supportive living environment. Physicians and nursing homes have also responded by opening offices and facilities within or near retirement new towns.

The aging population in new towns has prompted some residents to play an increasingly supportive role in their community. In one new town (Leisure World, California), resident groups have volunteered to look in on their aging neighbors, do their shopping, and even provide transportation. We also found that the increasingly aging population of one community was recognized by a local governmental unit which introduced a dial-a-ride service in the community. Finally, we have seen attempts by community builders to counteract the changing age structure of new towns by attracting younger retirees through advertisements and lower minimum age requirements.

The response of retirement villages to their aging populations, for the most part, has been similar to the responses of the retirement new towns. In many cases, however, the aging populations in villages have had to rely more on support services from the wider community than those aging residents of new towns. Villages tend to be less supportive, in part because they are less autonomous and more restrictive in their use of land for development of new, unplanned facilities. That is, unless land for facilities and/or programs for the future are contemplated and planned for at the inception of the retirement village project, the facilities and/or programs are unlikely to be provided at a later date.

Within retirement subdivisions, we were less likely to find dramatic changes in the average age of the population over time. As in the case of suburban developments everywhere, most residents move when their health deteriorates to the point where they require services that are not readily available. To a large extent, retirement subdivisions, which by definition provide limited services, cannot accommodate the elderly populations in their later years. No medical facilities exist, and in the case of trailer parks, the dwellings themselves become problematic for their occupants as they grow older. One exception, however, is Orange Gardens, where supportive housing with special design features that takes cognizance of older peoples' limited abilities was initially planned as part of the subdivision. In this instance, residents are able to remain as they age.

We have found our small sample of retirement residences to be moderately adaptive to the changing requirements of their aging population. One (Williams Memorial Residence) modified its rules to allow residents who needed private care to hire a helper or private nursing. Further, it relaxed its requirements with respect to the length of time people with disabilities could stay. We suspect, however, that most residences are not adaptive; they cannot provide for the changing needs of their aging populations.

The continuing care retirement center provides a highly adaptive living environment for the retirees who live there for extended periods. Within continuing care centers, a range of supportive services, including various forms of housing and levels of health care, are available to meet the changing needs of their residents. In some instances, we have seen the addition of more nursing beds and medical services as their residents have aged and the life support services become more sophisticated.

Growth in retirement communities. Retirement communities, as we have defined them, appear to grow in one of two ways. In one instance, they grow in size within the framework of a blueprint or Master Plan. The plan is either implemented instantaneously (within a 1- or 2-year period) or over an extended period of time. The second way in which retirement communities have grown is through incremental expansion. Incremental expansion occurs after the initial plan for the retirement community has been implemented. In other words, this form of growth was not anticipated at the time the actual plan was conceived, and usually results from the changing interests and needs of the residents and/or sponsors, including a desire to improve the quality of community life. In both instances, retirement community growth implies an increase in the number of residents and new physical structures, including facilities to support the residents.

The retirement new towns in our sample have each grown over an extended period of time according to a plan conceived at the inception of the community. In Sun City, Arizona, incremental expansion has occurred along with planned growth. Sun City West was started just prior to the completion of Sun City by its developer who was interested in meeting demand, far in excess of what was originally anticipated.

The retirement villages we examined also have grown over a period of time according to Master Plans. The Leisure Villages and Leisure World in Maryland have been built over a period of 10-15 years. At Hawthorne, Leisure Village, California, and Leisure World, Maryland, incremental growth is anticipated with the building of shopping centers on adjacent land.

The retirement subdivisions, retirement residences, and one of the continuing care centers were built within a relatively short period of time. The other continuing care centers in our sample experienced incremental growth since their inception. Otterbein Home, Presbyterian Home, and Sunny Shores have grown incrementally over a period of time, partly to meet the increasing demand for both nursing care and independent living units. Expansion has also been viewed by management as a means of generating new revenues to meet rising costs.

In a number of instances, we have seen where retirement community populations have increased more rapidly than the facilities needed to support the increase in the number of residents. While the timing and sequencing of growth has varied between and within classes of retirement communities, population increase usually precedes the provision of additional services and facilities. During some of our visits, we heard reports from long-term residents about deteriorating services, overcrowded facilities, more traffic and noise, and a perceived diminution of the quality of community life brought about by growth.

Population growth in new towns and retirement villages has also resulted in a decrease in the proportion of residents actively involved in the community affairs. For many long-term residents, the sense of being part of a "community" and the "feeling of belonging" have been lost. It is no longer possible for residents to know the names of all their neighbors as they once did. Similarly, it is impossible to remain active in every aspect of the community's social life and daily affairs. For others, however, growth, accompanied by deteriorating services and facilities, has presented a challenge, often met by greater involvement in community affairs. Participation in housing cooperatives, neighborhood groups, and planning organizations has given increasing numbers of retirement village and new town residents a voice in running their affairs.

While deteriorating community services brought about by growth have resulted in participation in local affairs by significant numbers of retirement community residents, others have responded by using the facilities and services outside the retirement community or moving to another location. In one place (Sun City Center), greater use has been made of nearby commercial and recreational facilities. In another, however (Leisure Village, California), the development of a new shopping center as part of the retirement community has reduced usage of shopping facilities outside the community.

Incremental growth of the continuing care centers has fulfilled a demand for this type of retirement living in communities where the centers are located. In some instances, however, growth of such centers, particularly coupled with an increasing number of elderly within the entire area, has placed public service demands on the host community. In Sunny Shores, Florida, for instance, local bus service was extended to the retirement community as a result of its expansion. A local shopping center also extended its bus service to the retirement community. For the most part, however, the growth of continuing care retirement centers has placed little burden on their host communities.

In general, we have found that local business and governmental units have responded positively to retirement community growth. Retirees are viewed as desirable members of the wider community, having spending power and few demands. Members of the local business community often view retirees as potential customers. In the case of large-scale new town and retirement villages, growth means increased tax revenues, with relatively little provision of new services. In most instances, we have found that the expansion of large-scale developments have been accompanied by privately owned facilities necessary to support their growing populations.

Changes in the surrounding environs. For the most part, the environs within which retirement communities are located have changed dramatically since the funding of the communities. Three types of changes have taken place. First, there were the developmental changes which can be seen on the ground. Most often, these were changes in land use. Second, there were changes in populations who lived in the surrounding area. Finally, there were changes in the goals and objectives of governmental units and land holders with respect to the use of neighboring land in the host community.

A major physical change experienced in the surroundings is new residental development, which takes place on formerly vacant or agricultural land. Such change has occurred at two of the retirement new towns (Sun City, Leisure World, California), near Leisure World, Maryland, and at the Leisure Villages in California and New Jersey. In one new town (Sun City Center) and one village (Hawthorne), the surrounding areas have remained virtually unchanged during the period of community development. In those instances where residential growth has taken place on adjacent land, it has often been accompanied by supportive commercial uses, medical services, and publicly developed recreational and cultural facilities, such as recreation centers, libraries, and parks. These new services and facilities have benefited retirement community residents to the extent that the facilities are used by the retirees. In some places (Leisure World, California, Sun City), new development means more people in the area which has been viewed by some residents as a dilution of their political power. In response, many have taken up the cause of incorporation as a way of retaining control over decisions such as the manner in which tax dollars are spent. Incorporation, however, has not taken place.

For some retirement village residents, an increase in the neighboring population is seen as contributing to rising crime rates and concomitantly as a threat to their retirement community. In response, the security at many villages has been tightened with the introduction of patrols, higher perimeter fences, and tighter control at entry gates. These changes have tended to isolate the communities and their residents from the surrounding area. In fact, residents in some of the places we visited reported greater insularity as a result of growth that has taken place around them.

The development of greater Bradenton was viewed as instrumental in upgrading of the Bradenton Trailer Park subdivision in order to improve its overall image. In another retirement subdivision (Orange Gardens), development in the surroundings precipitated more traffic along its norther edge. As a result, many of the boundary properties have been allowed to deteriorate. However, the desirability of this and other subdivisions has been enhanced by the growth of non-residential uses such as shopping on adjacent lands.

For the most part, few changes have taken place in the area surrounding one of the two retirement residences we visited (Williams Memorial Residence in Manhattan). At the other (Baptist Gardens), a portion of the Long Beach, California area had deteriorated and was in the process of being redeveloped. During the period of decline, neighborhood crime had increased and several businesses used by the elderly residents were closed. For example, restaurants patronized by the retirees closed because of the changing character of the neighborhood. This contributed to the expansion of the residence's meals program. The changing character of the neighborhood also resulted in increased security at the residence.

We have also seen where development plans for adjacent properties have been actively opposed by retirement community residents. In Leisure World, Laguna Hills, for example, many residents opposed the developer's proposal for adjacent land, anticipating its elimination of bridle paths used by residents. Similarly, a proposed industrial use near Hawthorne was successfully opposed by the developer and community residents. Hawthorne residents were also instrumental in blocking a proposal for the creation of a fire district that would have included their community and raised their taxes.

Rising costs. It is not surprising to find that retirement communities have experienced rapidly rising costs during the past decade. As a result of high interest rates, tight monetary policies, and, more generally, double-digit inflation, developers and sponsors have found it increasingly difficult to build and operate retirement communities. At the same time, the cost of living in retirement communities has increased with regularity over the years. In particular, rising home prices have made it more expensive for new retirees to move into several retirement communities, while the high cost of home maintenance has affected established residents. The costs of providing and using services has also increased dramatically. Under these conditions, we have seen a number of specific changes taking place within several of our retirement communities.

In the retirement new towns, developers have responded to rising costs by slowing the pace of new development. Whereas in the early phases of development continuous speculative building and rapid sales served as a marketing mechanism to attract prospective buyers, developers have tended to build more on demand in recent years. With limited demand resulting from a generally depressed economy, development has progressed at a much slower rate than before. At the same time, some developers of retirement new towns, such as Sun City and Leisure World, California, have attempted to attract higher socioeconomic groups by building bigger and better quality housing and recreational facilities. Other developers (Sun City Center, Leisure World, Maryland) have responded by increasing the density of development so as to build more than the originally contemplated number of dwelling units. In one new town (Leisure World, California), the developer's response to high building costs was a changeover from cooperative development to condominiums, which offered him more favorable financing. This changeover also limited the number of moderate income retirees who could afford to move into the community.

In efforts to reduce the operating costs incurred by providing services to its residents, several retirement new towns and retirement villages have raised their maintenance fees and charges for other services. In Leisure Village, California, for example, a fee-for-service policy has been adopted for maintenance services previously included in the monthly charge. In another attempt to reduce maintenance costs, Country Village Apartments has introduced low maintenance ground cover. User fees for golf courses and other recreation facilities have been imposed in some places to both reduce costs and usage. These charges are generally resented by segments of the population.

Similar developer responses to high costs have been reported in retirement villages. In the Leisure Villages, for example, larger units, designed to attract higher socioeconomic groups, have been built in recent years. Some services, such as local transportation (Leisure Village, California), have been eliminated, although arrangements have been made by the residents to assist the local transportation authority in servicing the community. In other retirement villages (Country Village), reduction in services and the concomitant increases in fees and rentals have been accompanied by programs aimed at helping the citizenry reduce energy costs. In Hawthorne, rental fees for residential lots have increased, but not as rapidly as the developers would like, because of ceilings written into the leases. Finally, some retirement villages have contracted services to private vendors (Leisure World, Maryland).

We noted that in part because of rising costs, the retirement villages have been less likely than new towns to adapt to the changing medical and other needs of their residents as they age. While it is costly to do so, developers of retirement villages are not geared toward building more than housing units and the basic services needed to support them. As we noted earlier, retirees in retirement villages, compared to those in new towns, are more likely to either move from the community or rely on outside services as their needs for medical care increase.

Subdivisions having a predominantly retirement population are less likely to be affected by inflation and increasing costs than retirement new towns and villages. The development process is not affected, since subdivisions tend to be built within a short period of time. Increasing costs, however, do have an impact on some of the retirees living in subdivisions. Many who are seasonal residents have difficulty in maintaining two homes, and will give up one or the other. If they do leave the retirement subdivision, they are likely to be replaced by younger families. Residents of retirement subdivisions have also experienced an increase in monthly fees and mobile home lot rentals as a result of inflation. In some instances, residents have banded together and assumed responsibility for the operation and maintenance of services within a subdivision. For example, in Trailer Estates in Florida, residents run the clubhouse and maintain shuffleboard courts and the marina.

As in the case of retirement subdivisions, the building of retirement residences has not been greatly affected by rising costs, since they are built at one stage. In terms of their operations, many have raised rents, and some have initiated programs of energy conservation and the use of relatively inexpensive labor as a way of dealing with rising operating costs. In one instance (Baptist Gardens), the mandatory use of the dining room was imposed on residents along with an increase in rents.

The problem of rising costs has affected continuing care retirement centers primarily with respect to medical services. In most centers, continuing care contracts have continuously been changed and their rates have increased over time, in part to cover the future medical needs of the applicants, but also to cover the older residents whose health care needs have been more expensive than originally anticipated. This process has resulted in higher fees and an attraction of a higher socioeconomic clientele. Similarly, continuing care centers have attempted to bring in wealthier as well as younger retirees by building and marketing independent housing units. This approach has been used at Otterbein Home, Presbyterian Home, and Sunny Shores Villas.

Changes in governance and management. Over time, we have seen movement toward increasing resident involvement in retirement community governance, including an increase in their decision-making powers. This change has most often occurred in the retirement new towns, villages, and subdivisions. In several new towns and retirement villages (Sun City, Leisure World, California, Leisure Village California, Leisure Village, New Jersey, Leisure World, Maryland), residents have tended to increase their involvement in decision-making matters as the community has moved through various phases of development. This is particularly true in places with cooperatives and condominiums, where governance is tied to ownership. Initially, control of community operations has rested with either the developers or a management company. As the population grew, the decision-making powers of the developer have shifted to the residents. The changeover sometimes resulted from management problems, but, most often, it occurred as a result of state condominium laws. In general, however, the developer has retained ultimate control over the community until he is ready to "close out" his building activity. However, even when development is in process, various resident groups have sought to influence the nature of future development or at least to advise the developer on the activities that might be undertaken so as to best serve the population.

Perhaps the most extreme example of increasing resident involvement in governance is the outright purchase of the retirement community by the residents themselves. This has most often occurred in subdivisions, in part because they are the least expensive type of retirement community to buy. For example, residents of the Trailer Estates mobile home park purchased the subdivision outright for $275,000 in 1971 and since then have governed it themselves. In another mobile home park in Sarasota, Florida, residents have followed the same course of action. Finally, the residents of Hawthorne, a retirement village, are currently negotiating the purchase of the community from the developer, the Colonial Penn Insurance Company.

While the trend toward increasing citizen involvement has been apparent in large retirement communities developed over time and owned by the residents themselves, citizen involvement has been less extensive and more advisory in continuing care centers, retirement residences, and those retirement subdivisions where the residents rent their dwellings. Participation has often been a response to decisions made by the owner or sponsor and has focused on operational matters rather than developmental issues. In fact, residents of these small retirement communities have had no decision-making power; under current forms of ownership, they are unlikely to play more than advisory roles in community affairs.

Conclusion

During the past 30 years, we have witnessed a phenomenal growth in housing and living arrangements for the elderly. The phenomenon of mass longevity has had a profound impact on the entire societal fabric, including a variety of responses to the changing housing and life-style needs of the elderly. We have seen that retirement communities are one example, albeit a small one, of this type of response. In this book, we have attempted to demonstrate why and how a broad-based multi-dimensional typology of retirement communities could provide insight into the characteristics and experiences of these communities. Such an approach is significant because each type of community from the new town to the continuing care retirement center is indicative of a different set of responses to the different needs of a heterogeneous retirement population. The changing nature of each community type over time has also differed. It is our hope that this analysis will lead to a better understanding of the relative strengths and weaknesses of the various types of retirement communities with respect to the varying needs, capabilities, and desires of older people.

References

Aldridge, C. Informal social relationships in a retirement community. *Marriage and Family Living,* 21:70-72 (1959).

Barker, M. *California Retirement Communities.* Berkeley, California: The Center for Real Estate and Urban Economics, Institute of Urban and Regional Development, University of California (1966).

Bultena, G.L., and Wood, V. The American community: Bane or blessing? *Journal of Gerontology,* 24: 209-217 (1969).

Burby, R.J., and Weiss, S.F. *New Communities U.S.A.* Lexington, Massachusetts: D.C. Heath (1976).

Burgess, E. (Ed.) *Retirement Villages.* Ann Arbor: Division of Gerontology, The University of Michigan (1961).

Duncan, C. J., Streib, C., LaGreco, A., and O'Rand, A.M. *Retirement communities: Their aging process.* Paper presented at the 31st annual meeting of the Gerontological Society, Dallas, Texas (November 1978).

Feldt, A.G., Hindert, T.T., and Vakalo, K. *A Directory of Retirement Communities in the U.S.* Ann Arbor: National Policy Center on Housing and Living Arrangements, College of Architecture and Urban Planning, The University of Michigan (1981).

Gottschalk, S.S. *Communities and Alternatives: An Exploration of the Limits of Planning.* New York: Halsted Press (1975).

Hamovitch, M.E., and Larson, A.E. *The retirement village.* Paper presented at the Institute for State Executives in Aging at the University of Southern California, Idyllwild Campus (February 1966).

Heintz, M.M. *Retirement Communities.* New Brunswick, New Jersey: The Center for Urban Policy Research, Rutgers-The State University of New Jersey (1976).

Hoyt, G.G. The life of the retired in a trailer park. *American Journal of Sociology,* 59:361-370 (1954).

Lawton, M.P., *Environment and Aging.* Monterey, California: Brooks-Cole (1980).

Lawton, M.P., Greenbaum, M., and Liebowitz, B. The lifespan of housing environments for the aging. *The Gerontologist,* 20:56-64 (1980).

Miller, A.H., Gurin, P., and Gurin, G. *Age consciousness and political mobilization of older Americans.* Paper presented at the 32nd annual meeting of the Gerontological Society, Washington, D.C. (November 1979).

Mumford, L. For older people—Not segregation but integration. *Architectural Record,* 119:193-197 (1956).

Newman, S.J. Housing adjustments of the disabled elderly, *Gerontologist,* 16:312-317 (1976).

Peterson, J.A., Hamovitch, N., and Larsen, A.H. *Housing Needs and Satisfactions of the Elderly.* Los Angeles: Ethel Percy Andrus Gerontology Center, University of California (1973).

Sherman, S.R. The choice of retirement housing among the well-elderly. *Aging and Human Development*, Vol. 2(1971).
Webber, I., and Osterbind, C.C. Types of retirement villages. In E. Burgess (Ed.), *Retirement Villages*. Ann Arbor: The University of Michigan (1961).